BREAST CANCER BE-ATTITUDES!

by
Sylvia Morgan Baker

FIVE LOAVES PRESS
an imprint of
SILAS PUBLISHING
Atlanta, Georgia

Published by Silas Publishing
An Imprint of Silas Interactive Multimedia, LLC
1154 Westchester Drive
Lilburn, GA 30047 USA

*Breast Cancer Be-Attitudes: Embracing God's Thoughts
from Diagnosis Through Recovery*

The information in this book is true and complete to the best of our knowledge. However, all recommendations are made without any guarantee on the part of the author, contributors, or Publisher, who also disclaim any libaility incurred in connection with the use of this data or specific details. In particular, all medical decisions regarding appropriate treatment for breast cancer and its sequelae should be made only after direct consultation with a licensed physician.

Silas Publishing titles are also available at discounts in bulk quantity for industrial or sales-promotional and fund-raising use. For details, contact the publisher at the address listed above.

PCN Data
Baker, Sylvia Morgan.
Breast Cancer Be-Attitudes: Embracing God's Thoughts
from Diagnosis through Recovery / Sylvia Morgan Baker.

ISBN: 0-9745094-1-8
Printed and Manufactured in the United States of America

Acknowledgments

The author and publisher gratefully acknowledge the following persons for graciously granting permission to use their work:

Mindy Rollins (mindyrella@hotmail.com) of A Fine View for all illustrations in this book.

Sheila Jane Holt for the poem "Grief"

Eugenia Benner for the poem "A Full Moon's Autumn Eve"

Gail Kunkel for "Ice pellets gently sprinkled…"

Karissa N. Baker, R.N., B.S.N., for "Humor Therapy"

Robin Grady, R.N., C.H.T., for "Counseling as an Adjunct to Cancer Treatment"

Daniel R.L. Baker, B.N.H.S., N.D., for "Detoxification: What, Why, & How"

Eric Wilson, C.M.T., N.C.T.M.B., for "Massage & the Healing Connection"

Dr. Melita Braganza, M.B.B.S., D.C.H., for "Radiotherapy & Breast Cancer"

Dr. N. Joseph Haroun, M.D., for "Chemotherapy"

Dr. Chris Wright, Ph.D., for "Tamoxifen the 'Wonder Drug'"

Table of Contents

Acknowledgments 3

Dedication. 7

Foreword. 11

Chapter 1: Breast Cancer Personified 15

Chapter 2: The Earth Quakes. 19

Special: Humor Therapy. 23

Chapter 3: Toughing it Out: Fight or Flight?. 25

Chapter 4: Lumpectomy Frumpectomy 31

Special: Counseling as an Adjunct to Cancer Treatment 37

Chapter 5: Teammates 39

Chapter 6: We are the Mentally Challenged 43

Chapter 7: Infrastructure Design: Your Support &
Cheerleading Section 47

Chapter 8: Kafka-esque Cancer 51

Chapter 9: The Haunted House. 57

Chapter 10: Finding the Purpose 63

Chapter 11: Mastectomies Double-Take. 67

Chapter 12: Recovery. 73

Special: Massage & the Healing Connection. 79

Chapter 13: Thanksgiving Approaches 81

Chapter 14: Dodging Dark & Dismal Days. 87

Chapter 15: Trial Blessings. 93

Chapter 16: Freedom. 99

Chapter 17: Freely You Have Received...Freely Give. 103

Chapter 18: How Can I Help Thee? Let Me Count the Ways! 105

Chapter 19: Alternative Medicine: Prevention & Nutrition 109

Special: Recipes 115

Special: Detoxification: What, Why, & How. 123

Special: Radiotherapy & Breast Cancer 125

Special: Chemotherapy 129

Special: Tamoxifen the "Wonder Drug" 131

References & Reading. 137

Cancer Resources 139

About the Author 141

Dedication

Grief
She surprised me
with her simplicity.
Nothing to read between the lines,
Nothing to call by another name.

She was soft and even kind:
She touched me with memories
That felt like your hand on my head,
Like your breath on my cheek.
You are gone
and
I miss you.

–Sheila Jane Holt

COLLEEN MUDGETT was my hero of faith, and the mother of my high school buddy, Diane. Diane and I attended Kennett High School in Conway, NH, and we both graduated in 1974. I was the school's number one "Jesus freak," and Diane was a close second. During those years, our school was having a spiritual revival, and a number of us kids would go to Bible studies at Diane's house on the weekends. Bible studies at Diane's were so much fun! Colleen and her husband Bozie (his real name is Frank, but he was "Bozie" to us) were always overjoyed to see us come in through the kitchen door. Colleen would hug us all, bake us cookies, and praise the Lord. The spirit in her home on those evenings was exuberant and joyful.

The Mudgett's home had a quaint attic room, with slanted ceilings and beautiful handcrafted quilts on the walls. This cozy room was a

New Hampshire experience all its own and offered that feeling of nostalgia and comfort that I have found only in New Hampshire homes to which I am partial. The gigantic antique trunk that was positioned at the foot of the bed was festooned with fabric, ribbons, and buttons. Colleen would pull out all the fabric and describe to Diane the woolen jumpers she would make for her, exclaiming, "Oh, Diane, this would be just great for you! What fabrics do you want?" Colleen was the most gifted craftsman I knew. She caned chairs, re-upholstered anything, and created exquisite drapes and clothing. There seemed to be nothing she couldn't do with her hands.

Just six years after Diane and I graduated from high school, in 1981, Colleen was diagnosed with Stage Three Breast Cancer. She courageously had a mastectomy and radiation, followed by nine months of chemotherapy. But by 1989, Colleen and her family were told that the disease was now considered terminal. But wonder of wonders, Colleen was still with us until February, 2004. Since 1989, she had radiation treatment seven more times in various areas of her body and was on Tamoxifen, a drug that blocks the effects of estrogen, for a number of years.

But the things that most impressed me about Colleen were her fierce determination; her absolute, unwavering faith in God; and her ability to find any excuse to keep on living. She was truly a lover of life itself as she embraced it boldly, much as she embraced us as teenagers. I'm not sure how many times Colleen was told it was the end of the road, but if a grandchild was about to get married, or she had to help someone with a project, well, she just had to keep going. Give her a phone call, and that would be enough to keep her enthusiastic for months. Her love for God was contagious. She found her greatest comfort, as she often said, "sitting at His feet or cradled in His arms, where I can touch the hem of His garment."

It had been twenty-two years since Colleen was diagnosed with Stage Three Breast Cancer. Three summers ago her ribs began to fracture and her family knew there was a new battle to fight. During her last few months, Colleen was at home with hospice care twice a week. She was secure in knowing that this battle was the Lord's, as II Chronicles 20:17 claims: "Ye shall not need to fight this battle: set yourselves, stand ye still, and see the salvation of the Lord with you." Colleen knew this full well.

Colleen recently crossed that divine divide and is now rejoicing in her new home, where she will be forever comforted as she rests "cradled in His arms." Her final words were fitting: She thanked God for His years of faithfulness and rejoiced that this part of her journey was opening doors to a bright and exciting eternity.

Thank you, Colleen, for the inspiration you have been to so many other breast cancer survivors. We love you!

Foreword

The hardness of simply being human and subject to physical limitations finds its contrast in the spiritual life within.

BEING DIAGNOSED with breast cancer is a most frightening experience. The initial analysis of my condition was quite different from my final diagnosis. My team of doctors and I progressed through numerous biopsies, mammograms, sonograms, a lumpectomy, a sentinel node dissection, and a few other procedures before I finally had conclusive findings. (Not to mention I was filled with daunting medical terminology.)

My cancer was in Stage I, the earliest detectable stage of breast cancer. The tumor was "T1," meaning it was over one centimeter but less than two centimeters, and the lumpectomy and sentinel node dissection revealed that the lymph node situation was "N0," meaning "no known metastasis to axillary nodes." They identified the cancer type as an "infiltrating ductal carcinoma," which is the most common type of breast cancer. The tumor was "stellate," meaning it was a star-shaped, not round. I learned that stellate tumors have a poorer prognosis than round tumors. This tumor type is also called "poorly differentiated." Full-body scans confirmed that my metastasis condition was "M0," meaning that there was no distant metastasis.

Other factors that led me to make my final treatment decisions included the discoveries of (a) additional areas of infiltrating ductal carcinoma (which nearly escaped detection by even the very best of radiologists, surgeons, and radiation oncologists) and (b) multiple areas of microcalcification in both breasts as well as "atypical intraductal hyperplasia."

Each of us will have unique situations that influence our own treatment plan for breast cancer. Being well-informed is a *critical factor* in making decisions that we won't regret later. So to help *you* stay informed I have included sections by noted doctors about treatment options, some nutritious (and delicious) recipes, and recommended books and resources. I hope these will help you as you progress toward healing.

Throughout my own life crisis, I found my greatest source of strength in God's Word. Knowing His thoughts towards me, I embraced them instead of allowing myself to ponder on fear and doubt. Embracing God's thoughts is an opportunity each of us can enjoy in this great gift called life. Defining God's thoughts is the challenge we face because in order to know His thoughts toward us we must identify His character through what He has told us about Himself. When our belief system rests securely in God's loving and merciful nature, we can move forward with confidence, ready to face the multi-faceted challenges of life while enjoying the beauty and meaning of each new day.

During times of trial the virtue and treasure of polished womanhood is our reward. We grow in refinement and strength of character, *one thought at a time*. We decisively embrace life, with no false assumptions about immortality or convoluted ideas about the meaning of our existence. The hardness of simply being human and subject to physical limitations finds its contrast in the spiritual life within. When the mirror's dust and residue is removed, we will see looking back at us a woman of strength and honor, wisdom and kindness.

Today's Scripture

"For the weapons of our warfare are not carnal but mighty in God for pulling down strongholds, casting down arguments and every high thing that exalts itself against the knowledge of God, bringing every thought into captivity to the obedience of Christ."

–II Corinthians 10:4-5 (NKJV)

Quote

"The truth is more important than the facts."

–Frank Lloyd Wright (1868-1959)

Prayer

Lord, help us to remain focused on
the goodness of Your character,
knowing that as we think about You–on purpose,
You will fight our battles for us!
May our thoughts be anchored
in the resting place of Your nature
in the midst of our troubling concerns.
We offer You praise.
Amen

Musical Selection

Concerto Cm Rv 199 For Violin/Strings I: Alleg

–Antonio Vivaldi (1678-1741)

Chapter 1
Breast Cancer Personified

Learning to harness our faith with God's thoughts is the key to victorious living amidst a monster storm.

IF YOU ARE a breast cancer patient, you need no introduction to me, because you know me well already. I'm just like you. I've had to face my fears, make tough decisions, knowing that I would have to live with them. I've had to withstand the cruelties of breast cancer treatments and the tiresome, endless treks to medical appointments. You and I have in common the unsettling feeling of our worlds shaken up, our schedules being out of control, and the keen awareness of our own human vulnerability.

When cancer strikes, it puts us all on even ground. Rich or poor, pretty or plain, waitress or CEO, it makes no difference. There is no escape route and the only special treatment we'll get is that which is sent from Heaven. Yes, we know each other in an intimacy that perhaps we had rather not, but because that is true, we can communicate more intuitively and meaningfully.

I was forty-five years old when I was diagnosed with breast cancer. That was twenty-three years after I married my outrageous husband, Dan. I say outrageous because his outgoing personality, his great sense of humor, his capacity for fun, and his spirituality definitely set him apart. Following an eclectic career path including teaching history in a Christian school, founding a church, starting a Christian school, and pioneering a number of business enterprises, he accepted a position as Headmaster at an urban school with a wonderfully diverse population in Baltimore, Maryland.

I had been working for the previous principal, so when Dan joined the school he was the new boy on my block! Currently I serve as the Elementary Principal and Director of Curriculum Development. Dan and I enjoy the ultimate blessing of our two wonderful kids, Karissa, twenty-two, and Daniel, twenty, who brighten our lives with unspeakable joy.

Our lives have not been perfect, but they have been perfectly blessed. Dan was with me for every doctor's appointment, blood test, X-ray, biopsy, and all those surgeries. His support was and remains an extension of God's boundless, never-ending compassion and grace. His life speaks clearly of divine resources and bears witness of God's presence.

In the pages to follow, I will share my story with you and explore the mighty mystery of faith. Let's face it; it's devastating to think that God would allow us to suffer. When one learns that he or she has cancer, the relevance of salvation is often questioned.

I never considered that one in eight Christian women would need to deal with breast cancer! Somehow I assumed that I would be exempt from the list of women that breast cancer would strike. I found the breast cancer challenge to be the ultimate test in facing my fears and addressing my faith. In the panic stages of cancer, faith is like a train that has run off the tracks—you just can't get your hands on it; faith seems to slip away.

Learning to harness our faith with God's thoughts is the key to victorious living in the midst of a monster storm. Psalm 119:88 says, "Quicken me after thy lovingkindness, so shall I keep the testimony of my mouth." Establishing confidence in God's nature so that we can orientate our thoughts toward healing is central to relaxation in times of trial.

I like to refer to God's provision as the "No-Fault Divine Insurance Plan." I likened my breast cancer to an unexpected automobile accident. It was no one's fault. And God's insurance plan would cover me and, in the end, I would have a new vehicle, in spite of all the hassle with paperwork and procedures.

The search for meaning in breast cancer inevitably emerges as we progress through the many phases of treatment and healing. Embracing God's thoughts about suffering brings us peace and reassurance that He is at work within us and through our suffering. This brightens our world! Learning to speak the truth about God's faithfulness enables us to love our lives, even in tumultuous times. I Peter 3:10 says, "For he that will love life and see good days, let him refrain his tongue from evil and his lips that they speak no guile." Embracing faithful thoughts energizes us and those around us to hold on to hope, with confident expectation for better days ahead.

Years ago, our pastor's wife would sing "The Darker the Night, the Brighter the Light Shines." It was her theme song. I never heard her sing anything else. She slowly lost her life to leukemia, but she also saw the eternal light of Christ shining brightly in darkness.

I can promise you this much–the cancer journey will open windows of hope and joy and doors of opportunity for unexpected surprises and blessings. Just as God has promised, "I will give you the treasures in darkness and hidden riches of secret places" (Isaiah 45:3, NKJV).

Climate Control

With sun pushing up over the bay
I listen to the news to discover–
What will the climate be today,
Sunshine–or clouds that hover?

My preference would be sunshine
With a gentle breeze from the north,
Bringing a fresh temperature divine–
Then I would frolic in summer's mirth.

Mostly cloudy is not too bad
Since cooler weather brings relief.
Rain, however spoils my plans
And thunderstorms unearth my inner grief.

I cannot control the climate
of mid-Atlantic summer's weather pattern.
But I can muse on heavenly views of
egrets flying low in Harford Glen.

Today's Scripture

"For in that He Himself has suffered, being tempted, He is able to aid those who are tempted."

–Hebrews 2:18 (NKJV)

Quote

"Whether you think that you can, or that you can't, you are usually right."

–Henry Ford (1863-1947)

Prayer

Father, may Your presence
during our time of suffering fill us
and overflow so that we reflect grace
and Your goodness to others in our path.
We rejoice in trusting you:
Your comfort is perfect.
Let us find rest in
Your merciful embrace.
Amen

Musical Selection

Aria

–George Frideric Handel (1685-1759)

Chapter 2
The Earth Quakes

The idea that I could, with conscious effort, change my thinking by choosing my thoughts grew from an idealistic concept to a lifestyle in a short span of time.

YOU WILL PROBABLY never forget where you were when you first heard the sinister "C" word with your name attached to it. It took me several weeks before I could actually say the word "cancer" without wincing. I was in my office working one day when my doctor called and told me that I needed to see a surgeon. I couldn't imagine why. I wasn't prepared for that. And maybe nothing can shield you from the shock of learning that cancer has grown in your body.

A short time later, the phone rang again. We were at home that evening, and Dan and I had been through the whole nerve-wracking "We're pretty sure it's cancer" ordeal, and now we were going to know for sure exactly what my diagnosis was. When the doctor asked me to put Dan on the line, too, my heart sank. I was on one phone and Dan was on the other, listening. My surgeon told us that the "stereotactic biopsy" had revealed a one centimeter malignant tumor. Four of the six biopsied sections, he said, revealed "well-differentiated, infiltrating duct carcinoma." The tumor was "estrogen receptor positive."

Somehow, with my mind a befuddled cloud, I understood that "well-differentiated" was a good thing, and that "estrogen receptor positive" could be helpful for treatment. But I also knew that "infiltrating" meant aggressive.

Nothing shatters your nerves and numbs your mind like the horrible news that you are suffering from a potentially fatal illness. The mysterious truth of facing your own mortality, suddenly unmasked, feels much like sinking in quicksand with a cement truck headed toward you at the same time.

We all know that we will die one day. But we God-pursuing Christians, whose spirits are continually quickened with *auto-pilot faith thoughts*, rest in God's abiding love. We have sipped eternal waters, so we go about our lives relaxed about the whole "death issue." We rely on our good Father to deliver on His promise of eternal life. But somewhere in the background of our consciousness is that nagging awareness of death's dreaded impasse. In the midst of life's routines, trials, celebrations, disappointments, and expectations, the corruption of the physical body is a subject we avoid as diplomatically as we can. And there it was, for me, staring me in the face.

A few days after that phone call, I awoke to the wonderful discovery that neither the quicksand nor the truck had killed me yet. I was still here in my earthen vessel–a body of death still breathing life. The initial shock of breast cancer had begun to subside, and I was confronted with the reality that I was in a quandary from which there was no imminent escape. Through some God-given enlightenment, it dawned on me that while the news of having cancer would require a sober, proactive response, the old news of God's faithfulness was still true!

With my daily routines rapidly and dramatically changing, I had a choice to make. I could focus on the new *bad* news or focus on the old *good* news. I determined to make a deliberate decision to hold fast to my faith, not wavering, knowing that our God is faithful, as we learn in Hebrews 10:23.

My thought-life was the perfect place to exercise faith in God's provisions. The notion that I could, with conscious effort, change my feelings by choosing my thoughts went from an idealistic concept to a *lifestyle* in a very short span of time. By thinking specifically with God's Word and what He tells us about Himself, my *gigantic* details quickly resumed their miniscule stature. The fact is: We are here today, hopefully not gone to heaven by tomorrow, so our best option is to live in the present, applying wonderful attitudes of grace and goodness for today.

I've heard it said that yesterday has passed away, tomorrow isn't here yet, but *today*, this moment, is ours to capture if we will only choose to abide in God's thoughts toward us. Yes, Jeremiah 29:11 is clear, "For I know the thoughts that I think toward you; thoughts of peace and not of evil, to give you an expected end."

When we choose to let expectation team up with hope, we are able to laugh at the ridiculous, believe in the impossible, dream of the future, and delight in the smallest joys of every day. I try to make it my habit to *imagine the miraculous*, as Anne Sullivan must have when she committed herself to tutoring the "unteachable" Helen Keller. Only expectation teamed up with hope could have discovered the brilliance that lay where mortal eyes could never see.

With such courageous thinking, we are sure to win our battles!

Today's Scripture

"But the meek shall inherit the earth: and shall delight themselves in the abundance of peace."

–Psalm 37:11 (KJV)

Quote

"When you do the common things in life in an uncommon way, you will command the attention of the world."

–George Washington Carver (1864-1943)

Prayer

We thank You Lord, for the provision
of Your living Word. May we take the time today
to read, ponder, and meditate about
the life-giving promises You have made to us.
We thank You that You are an immutable God.
We thank You that You cannot change
Your mind about how You think towards us.
With joy may we approach today, with deep,
residual comfort that comes from choosing

to consider Your thoughts about us.

Amen

Musical Selection

Pamphlets (Waltz)

–Johann Strauss II (1825-1899)

Humor Therapy

By Karissa N. Baker, R.N., B.S.N.

LAUGHTER IS a momentary release from the intensity of what otherwise might be overwhelming. A sense of humor can help you overlook the unattractive, tolerate the unpleasant, cope with the unexpected, and smile through the unbearable. Emotions modulate the activity and effectiveness of the immune cells although the emotions do not directly protect the body from insult or infection.

Our interpretation of stress is not dependent solely on an external event, but also on our perception of the event and the meaning we give it. How we perceive and respond to an illness will determine it to be a threat or a challenge for us. While we cannot control events in our world, we can control how we view the events and we can choose our emotional response. Humor can positively affect us in the following ways:

- Reduces stress
- Boosts immunity by lowering serum cortisol levels and increasing activated T-lymphocytes, Natural Killer cells, and T-cells
- Relieves pain
- Decreases anxiety
- Stabilizes mood
- Rests the brain
- Enhances communication
- Releases tension in the diaphragm and relieves pressure on liver and other internal organs

Remember, the body grows fat from joy and thin from sadness. So go ahead and have some fun. After all, it's good for you!

Chapter 3
Toughing it Out:
Fight or Flight?

I encourage you to carefully consider the fact that cancer usually offers its boxing match just once, although you may have several rounds in the ring if you take the challenge.

Say Naught the Struggle Naught Availeth
Say not the struggle naught availeth,
The labour and the wounds are vain,
The enemy faints not, nor faileth,
And as things have been they remain.
If hopes were dupes, fears may be liars;
It may be, in yon smoke conceal'd,
Your comrades chase e'en now the fliers,
And, but for you, possess the field.
For while the tired waves, vainly breaking,
Seem here no painful inch to gain,
Far back, through creeks and inlets making,
Comes silent, flooding in, the main.
And not by eastern windows only,
When daylight comes, comes in the light;
In front the sun climbs slow, how slowly!
But westward, look, the land is bright!

–Arthur Hugh Clough (1819-1861)

WHEN THE GOING gets tough, the tough get going. This quote might have been coined by Joseph Patrick Kennedy, or football coach Knute Rockne, or even by the dear one, Mother Teresa. Regardless where it came from, it is true! If you have been diagnosed with breast cancer, you surely do have it tough right now. So it's time to get going, channelling your energies toward healing. But before you do, take a moment to offer a prayer of thanksgiving that your cancer has been found and that you are in very capable hands–*God's*.

After seven years of suspicious mammograms and return visits to radiologists for one more picture, "just to be sure," I still didn't know what "calcification" meant. The term had always seemed innocent enough to me. Thus, I chose to dismiss it as a possible blessing from drinking too much milk as a child. Or maybe it was a sign that I wouldn't get osteoporosis because I had extra "calci" something in my bazooms! Well, you were probably better informed than I was, if indeed you had a series of suspicious mammograms. As for me, though, I really enjoyed having my head in the sand with a case of the OC–the Ostrich Complex. Avoidance afforded me the benefit of having one less thing to worry about because, really, I didn't have time to be sick. And who has time to research things that are not supposed to be a problem?

Looking back, I find it almost incomprehensible that no radiologist ever explained to me that calcifications are a common precursor to breast cancer. Had I known that sooner, I believe I would have made some lifestyle changes to take some preventive measures against breast cancer.

I hope you have made a conscious and deliberate decision to put on the boxing gloves and beat up on the cancer. I hope, too, that *your* faith in God speaks to you of God's faith in *you*. God understands fully the difficult and unpleasant experiences you may encounter if you decide to fight for your life. No one can fight this very private fight for you. You must make the commitment to yourself and for yourself. Now it's just you and God, baby!

While you must fight the fight yourself, the comfort of others' support and company is so meaningful during this time because the fight is so intensely personal. You need the support and company of others as you fight your good fight against the disease.

The decision to do whatever it takes to save your life may come grudgingly–as no one wants to suffer. Yet Christ is our example especially in this area. He suffered as no one ever has, knowing all the while that the outcome of His pain would mean eternal life for humankind. Your decision, too, will mean sacrifice. It may mean surgery, painful recovery periods, chemotherapy, radiation, nausea, hair loss, and other unpleasant *but temporary* experiences.

For some, it may mean a lumpectomy only–if you are fortunate enough to have been diagnosed very early with a small, non-aggressive tumor. I encourage you to carefully consider the fact that cancer usually offers its boxing match just once, although you may have several rounds in the ring if you take the challenge. I recall the games my son's baseball team won because the opposing team forfeited by not showing up. Those victories were harder to celebrate. I knew right away that I wanted to show up for this fight, but there was no way I could possibly have known where that commitment would lead.

Since you can be pretty sure that some kind of treatment plan will be suggested upon diagnosis, now is a great time to become an ECBR–an Effective Breast Cancer Researcher!

If you're going to *consume* cancer treatments, become an informed consumer:

- Go to the library and read everything you can get your hands on, because time is passing and you will need to make serious decisions in a timely manner.

- Get thee to the Web and browse!

- Compare and contrast what nationally recognized breast cancer specialists have to say about the specific kind of cancer you are diagnosed with.

- Ask questions. Be a nuisance if you need to!

- Learn about your options.

- Make notes.

Proverbs 11:14 says, "In the multitude of counselors there is safety." How true. There is nothing worse than undermining your efforts with second-guessing. You must claim ownership of each treatment decision that you will make. Sometimes ignorance is indeed bliss, but when it comes to breast cancer it isn't. Knowledge can only help you in your fight.

When I let go of my fear of learning what "calcification" really meant and started researching it, I was empowered to make some very difficult and heart-wrenching decisions. In the final analysis, when I had gathered and processed all the information, I still had to wait on God for His direction and specific guidance for each step of the cancer treatment pathway. There is nothing pleasant about breast cancer treatment aside from God's presence, but if you patiently endure the healing process, you will find peace and even joy.

When you learn all that's entailed in your breast cancer treatment plan, you may be tempted to get discouraged. Remember this: If you choose to embrace God's thoughts to cast down fearful imaginations, contentment will find a home in your soul. Exchanging fear and discouragement for a tough, warrior attitude did a lot to transform me from a scared, wimpy whiner to a tough, deliberate, and bold cancer fighter. So go ahead, tough one, start fighting!

Today's Scripture

"Blessed be the LORD my strength, which teacheth my hands to war, and my fingers to fight."

–Psalm 144:1 (KJV)

Quote

"We are not retreating–we are advancing in another direction."

–General Douglas MacArthur (1880-1964)

Prayer

Father, we ask You to give us the courage
to take steps toward healing, no matter how
daunting they may appear.
Grant us the courage to stay objective,
the determination to gather information,

and the persuasion to move quickly.
Please Father, we ask You to shine Your countenance
of favor on us as we act
humbly yet decisively and bravely.
Amen

Musical Selection

Suite Bb–Prelude

–Marin Marais (1656-1728)

Chapter 4
Lumpectomy Frumpectomy

---

*The stubbornness of a mood is often just displaced anxiety;
when we're dealing with multiplying cancer cells, it's the peace
we need multiplied, not the stress.*

WITH MUCH PRAYER and magnanimous peace, I followed the advice of my surgeon and scheduled a lumpectomy and sentinel node dissection for September 4. Nerves all a-jitter, I gladly inhaled the anesthesia, relieved to be delivering my consciousness to God and my tumor to the surgeon. When I regained consciousness, I found myself sick and vomiting from the anesthesia. The drain hanging from under my right arm reminded me why I was there, in the hospital, as Dan's anxious face belied his words of comfort.

A lumpectomy and sentinel node dissection are considered outpatient procedures, so as soon as I could quit vomiting and pull myself together to get to the car, wheelchair transport and all, we headed for home. Once there, I dragged myself up the stairs, proclaiming to anyone within earshot that this had been the worst day of my life!

Little did I know what was coming. Fortunately, only our dog Dakota was there to hear me, as Karissa and Daniel were not yet home from their college classes. Bandage fiddling and drain manipulating aside, in retrospect I don't think I suffered that badly from the lumpectomy. Within a few days I was feeling much better, although not much better about myself. When I looked in the mirror, I met "frump-woman," the side-effect of lumpectomy.

I had exchanged the lump for the frump! Oh, dear. Where was my makeup? When could I shower? I searched frantically and fruitlessly to find the old me who was hanging out backstage somewhere, waiting for the next act.

We humans are unpredictable, so given any set of circumstances we're not sure what to expect—the good, the bad, or the *ugly*! The point is that *unless we make a conscious decision* to live in the new, to focus on the positive, and to "be renewed in the spirit of our mind" (Ephesians 4:23) our old, natural way of thinking will squelch our new spiritual way of thinking and seeing that comes from embracing God's thoughts about us. After my encounter with frump-woman, I decided to stay away from mirrors for a couple of days, but whenever frump-woman's image would pop into my mind, I would replace her with more pleasant images. Sometimes I would picture a yard-full of dogwoods, azaleas, and cherry blossoms. Other times I would call up the comforting faces of my husband, my children, my parents, my siblings.

When we *feel* unlovely because we're sick or just plain sick of it all, we must exercise God's compassion for ourselves. Placing a priority on love of self and others liberates us to embrace our ridiculous circumstances with the poise and honor of royalty. We are indeed royalty, so why not act the part. If it doesn't come to you naturally, then just "faith it" for a while. Pretending to be loved by God when not feeling or looking especially loveable is a lot more fun than moping around the house, absorbed in self-pity and looking in mirrors at a project in progress. Soon your faith confessions will work their way into your thinking patterns and you will find yourself enjoying the company of frump-woman after all.

Moods can be stubborn things! And often this stubbornness is caused by displaced anxiety. When we see it for what it is—anxiety— we can release it to God, instead of internalizing it and multiplying the stress so that it comes out as an unshakable mood, or image of frump-woman. And when we're dealing with multiplying cancer cells, it's the peace we need multiplied, not the stress!

A few days after the lumpectomy, my surgeon called with the lab results. There was good news and bad news. Which did I want to hear first? Hoping to focus on the good news, I took the bad news first. The bad news was that the lab results showed that there was greater "mitotic activity" than originally indicated by the stereotactic biopsy. There was "nuclear pleomorphism," whatever that was, and rather than being well differentiated, the tumor was poorly differentiated. The cancer was infiltrating, meaning that it was aggressive, and was scattered throughout a number of areas. That definitely sounded like bad news.

So what was the good news? The good news was that the sentinel node dissection had come back clean, meaning there was no indication that the cancer had spread through the lymph nodes and into my blood stream. *Hallelujah!* Brief sigh of relief–I had been holding my breath. *Joyous interlude!* With negative nodes I felt that I had the advantage in the ring. At least I had won this round. With the results of my lab report and oncology statistics, my team of doctors was in a better position to define treatment options for me.

I recall that I spent a good deal of time in the library the first week after my primary care physician told me I had cancer. As I was researching breast cancer the word "statistic" kept popping up. In my panicked state, I was convinced that my very best prognosis would be to survive for five years. That's what those *statistics* said. What I didn't know then was that the studies typically stop after five years. Who were the mothers, sisters, aunts, and grandmothers who had provided the statistics? Would I be a statistics provider? I didn't want the job! The truth is that breast cancer survivors may live very long and healthy lives, and the statistics, used rightly, can be very useful in helping women make educated treatment decisions for the various stages of breast cancer.

My medical oncologist, the warm and reassuring Dr. Madhu Chaudhry of Greater Baltimore Medical Center (GBMC), recommended that I begin chemotherapy treatment soon, perhaps with tamoxifen for five years. Usually a lumpectomy is followed by radiation therapy first, and then chemotherapy. Early mammograms had revealed moderate density in the left breast and mild asymmetry with no dominant mass. Another mammogram confirmed that there was no mass on the left breast, though there did appear to be more density than in previous mammograms and several areas of calcifications were identified. I was told to be thankful. I was.

I was still nervous about that left breast, though. My surgeon referred me to a specialist–a radiation oncologist at GBMC–to discuss radiation. He assured me that radiation would take care of any "remaining concerns." Remaining concerns? That phrase stuck with me, nagging me, as the last thing I wanted were any *remaining concerns*. My goal was to get through this phase of my life and live free from breast cancer, because I knew that aging in itself would bring challenges.

That evening after the sun set we were tired. Tired of thinking about medical terminology, tired of having it refer to me, tired of the worry, tired of wondering. So we pulled our pillows together and prayed for no "remaining concerns."

Today's Scripture

"Favour is deceitful, and beauty is vain: but a woman that feareth the LORD, she shall be praised."

–Proverbs 31:30 (KJV)

Quote

"Obstacles are those frightful things you see when you take your eyes off your goal."

–Henry Ford (1863-1947)

Prayer

Lord, help me to see You looking back at me
in the mirror as I learn to focus on my inner man
more intently than my outer image.
Cause me to receive words of edification
with the sincerity and purity
with which they are offered.
Let me rest in Your love,
knowing I am complete in You.
Amen

Musical Selection

Ich Liebe Dich (I Love You)

–Edvard Grieg (1843-1907)

Counseling as an Adjunct to Cancer Treatment

By Robin Grady, R.N., C.H.T.

CHRISTIAN COUNSELING is an effective tool for the cancer patient in dealing with the devastation of the disease, cancer pain, and the healing process. Through guided imagery and visualization, negative thought patterns that impede healing can be released. They can be replaced by the restorative power of God's thoughts. The counselor can help the patient refocus on this healing power, thus helping the patient to experience inner peace and strength in the face of any adversity. The mind-body connection is as real as God's Word, for we read in Proverbs 23:7, "For as a man thinketh in his heart, so is he."

It is important to discuss your belief system with your counselor before beginning sessions to ensure that your values and perspectives are complementary. By re-training our thought patterns to reflect all of who we were created to be, we can maximize the spiritual, mental, and the physical health that is within our reach.

Robin Grady is a registered nurse and a clinical therapist certified by the International Medical and Dental Hypnotherapy Association. Her study has focused on Biblical application in helping hurting people find meaning and purpose. She maintains a private practice in Bel Air, Maryland.

Chapter 5
Teammates

Sometimes a simple miscommunication can spiral downward quickly when we are under much pressure to move speedily and aggressively against the cancer.

THE WORD TEAM usually makes us think of the qualities of a championship ball club or a celebrated orchestra. Team members work together, communicating with one another for the good of the whole. When *I* think of a team I have something slightly different in mind. I think of a team of inspired medical professionals who work together to achieve one goal–what is best for you, their patient.

Having a great medical team in your corner will promote in you an attitude of confidence and assurance. When doctors collaborate effectively, they will ensure that your treatment and healing plan progresses as quickly, yet tranquilly, as possible. And you are the one who benefits!

I was truly blessed with a wonderful team of doctors. They not only treated me with respect and professionalism but they were congenial to each other. At no time did I sense that one doctor was out of the loop and lacking accurate, up-to-date information on my medical status. This helped give me a sense of stability and security–which are two things breast cancer patients sorely need. Your team of health care providers will probably look much like mine and include your primary care physician, a medical oncologist, a surgeon, a plastic surgeon, a radiation oncologist, and a host of other medical staffers such as nurses and X-ray technicians.

Shortly after I got my diagnosis, two of my close friends found out that they, too, had breast cancer. It seemed that once I had breast cancer, everyone I met had breast cancer or knew someone who did. I spoke to many women about their medical and healing experiences, and many were overjoyed with their team of doctors who were willing to put aside schedules, personal preferences, and sometimes even family vacations for their patient's good.

I have talked to a few breast cancer patients, however, who were not so pleased with their team. In some cases, the women felt uncomfortable with their doctors and found it to be a very distressing experience. Many of the women shared a concern over the length of time they had to wait before a surgery could be scheduled. Some did not have access to doctors when they really needed to speak with them. In some cases, the women felt that their doctors did not explain things to them comprehensively enough, and, worse, some assumed a condescending attitude towards them. I am delighted to say that I had none of those disconcerting experiences with my wonderful team of medical professionals.

If you are not so blessed and find yourself frustrated with your doctors, there are a couple of things you can do. First, schedule a conference to try to work through the problem. Sometimes a simple miscommunication can spiral downward quickly when we are under a lot of stress to move speedily and aggressively against the cancer. If you are not married and usually go to your appointments alone, perhaps you could ask a friend or loved one to attend the meeting with you to offer an objective perspective on the relationship and possibly help to clarify your concerns by posing questions differently than you might.

Second, if after discussing your concerns with your doctor, you are still not comfortable with the outcome, then please get another doctor. I've been told that there is currently a shortage of oncologists, but the shortage is not so great that you cannot shop around. Your confidence in and comfort with your team is critical. The last thing anyone needs when facing life or death decisions is a relationship that causes additional stress—especially with someone who plays such an important role as a doctor.

Another problem that can bring stress is not being able to get appointments scheduled promptly. This one is not the fault of your team of doctors. You will likely need to have bone scans, MRIs, blood work, and many other such tests. When you can't get an appointment within the time frame that your doctor recommends it can be very frustrating. I recall showing up for a scheduled bone scan, only to find out that the secretary had scheduled me for an entirely different procedure. It was clearly an office error, but I was told I could not get the scan for another week, which caused me immediate anxiety. When things like this happened, I found it helpful to insist on speaking to the manager on duty. In the misscheduled bone scan case, I explained my point of view. It so happened that I was particularly frustrated that day, and I reminded the manager that she was overlooking an office error that could well alter the outcome of my cancer treatment by delaying a needed treatment. I may have been exaggerating, but it may very well have been true. I suggested that the manager either ask someone to work overtime or send me to another facility. It turned out that I was able to get the scan the following morning, which spared me further stressful delays.

Your journey through breast cancer treatment will at times be stressful, but remember this: Because God is on your side you need not despair in your pursuit of health and healing. His unfailing love for you will cause even unpleasant things to work for your benefit. This assurance is given us in Romans 8:38-39: "For I am persuaded that neither death nor life, nor angels, nor principalities, nor powers, nor things present, nor things to come, nor height, nor depth, nor any other created thing shall be able to separate us from the love of God which is in Christ Jesus our Lord." When the schedule may not follow our expectations, our best option is to trust that God has us covered and ensures our best outcome.

Today's Scripture

"Counsel is mine, and sound wisdom; I am understanding, I have strength."

–Proverbs 8:14 (NKJV)

Quote

"When you can't trace God's hand, you can trust God's heart."

–Charles Haddon Spurgeon (1834-1892)

Prayer

I thank you for Your example of complete
trust in the Father's plan.
You knew Your Father's heart so well.
Help me to take the next step before me,
knowing you have lead each physician,
consultant, lab technician and nurse
who has brought me this far.
I praise you for Your omniscience
that sees the end from the beginning–
in You I find my peace as
the sun sets behind my mountains.
Amen

Musical Selection

Fantasie-Impromptu C#M Op. 66

–Frederic Chopin (1810-1849)

Chapter 6
We Are The Mentally Challenged

> *If we're not diligent in our spiritual fitness regimen
> we will lose focus on God's thoughts.*

HAVE YOU ever started an exercise program the the best of intentions, only to have it last about three weeks or, perhaps, three days? Maybe you're a whole lot more disciplined than I am in that area and know firsthand the benefits of repetitive, consistent exercise. I must admit that my own knowledge about it is secondhand. It comes from seeing our son, Daniel, reap the wonderful benefits of his disciplined exercise and fitness routine. Regular exercise improves muscle tone and cardiac health and benefits the whole body.

Exercising the spirit gets benefits and results, too. *But how is it done? How do we exercise our spirit?* Well, it's so simple that we forget to do it, much as I forget to pick up the weights for working out my arms. A spiritual fitness program requires some simple steps that lead to spiritual and psychological fitness.

- Step one involves making a mental note of God's goodness several times a day. Recall the times God has been faithful to you, even in little things.

- Step two involves setting aside some time each day to meditate.

I didn't have much expendable time before cancer, but after I was diagnosed I had even less because I had to jump through medical hoops galore. Finding divine serenity in the cancer treatment web is not as difficult as it seems at first. Meditation on Christ does not require a special time and place set aside to focus–although that luxury would be wonderful. Divine meditation is simply the process of selectively choosing our thoughts according to the Word of God. Negative thoughts are never in short supply. If we don't dream them up ourselves, someone else is sure to offer them. Pessimistic thought-patterns run downhill and contradict the hope that pleasant thoughts bring. I love the challenge of finding a good report. It seems the whole world is determined to give bad reports!

Philippians 4:8 challenges us to "think on things that are true, honest, just, pure, lovely, and of good report." Anything of virtue, anything of praise, is a good thing to focus our thoughts on. *But what about dealing with reality and facing the facts?* While it is a human fact that you have cancer, it is a divine fact that God is faithful. Verbalizing faith really does help dispel negative fungus in the mind. Have you ever tried it? I challenge you to try it. The next time a bad reporter is in your life-space, try mentioning how thankful you are that God is so good. Everyone's spirits will pick up, but most importantly, your own.

If we're not diligent in our spiritual fitness regimen we will lose focus on God's thoughts. Staying focused and reflecting on good reports was vital for me while my life was revolving around a bad report. Pondering God's goodness and the hope found there freed my soul to soar above the threat of illness. If you have been diagnosed with breast cancer, there is a battle to fight–on two fronts. Equal to, and perhaps *greater than*, the physical battle is the battle that will be fought in your mind. You cannot whimsically excuse random negative thought-patterns; for they grow fast like weeds and will choke out the spiritual fruit that you have cultivated.

I challenge you to become a champion at embracing God's thoughts so that you will be able to cast down vain, empty, negative imaginations and pick up a good report! Your capacity for mental, physical, and spiritual healing will equal your capacity for meditation and solitude. Some experts contend that the mind and body are so intimately connected that you cannot truly distinguish one from the other. How much more effective we will be in our fight against breast cancer if we learn to discipline our thoughts and speak to our bodies with words of encouragement and healing. With the right thoughts in place, we are better equipped to communicate our concerns, our needs, and our progress with our team of family, friends, and medical staff. Exercise your mind with God's thoughts!

Today's Scripture

"Blessed be the Lord, who daily loadeth us with benefits, even the God of our salvation. Selah."

–Psalm 68:19 (KJV)

Quote

"Men are not disturbed by things, but the view they take of things."

–Epictetus (55-135 A.D.)

Prayer

Lord, we pray that anger, depression, or anxiety
will not overcome us with confusion,
but that through concentration on goodness,
we will overcome with peace that overcomes
our limited understanding of temporary situations.
Grant us Your presence, beginning with
our thought lives. We release our inner fears
and offer you thanks and praise.

Amen

Musical Selection

Horn Concerto Eb Kv 417 111: Rondo
–Wolfgang Amadeus Mozart (1756-1791)

Chapter 7
Infrastructure Design: Your Support & Cheerleading Section

If you live alone, or if the people you live with are difficult to bare your heart to, then I pray for God to send you someone with whom you can honestly share your needs.

BEFORE YOU can really get down to business battling the cancer and starting treatments, you will want to share the news with your loved ones. Telling our children that I had breast cancer was one of the hardest things I had to do–especially since my diagnosis was so unexpected. At that point I didn't know the full extent of my illness, so Dan and I were able to give Karissa and Daniel a lot of hope that things would turn out fine after a simple surgery. No, we told them, I would not lose my breasts and probably wouldn't even need chemotherapy. I was *one of the lucky ones* who had such a very simple problem that you could hardly even call it cancer. Clearly, I was still hoping for the best scenario!

I had always thought that if I ever got really sick, I would tell only the members of my immediate family and thus manage to slip quietly through the illness and get it over with. I vowed I would keep it "a minor detail." I know that some people associate shame with illness and others take it as a personal failure. I don't think these are true, but, nevertheless, deciding whom you want or need in your inner circle is a very personal matter. For me, I needed to grow into each treatment decision without a lot of well-intentioned, but sometimes misinformed, people coaching me. Owning your decisions does not mean, however, that you will not need support. Trust me, you will need tons of support to get through this season in your life.

You will need a great deal of practical help, so if you are one of those fiercely independent people who hates for other people to help you with anything, I'd suggest that you take a short vacation from your temperament and let some good-hearted people become helpers of your joy.

If you are not well networked with a church or other social community, then you might want to contact the American Cancer Society. There are many volunteers who would love to help drive you to appointments, bring a meal by your home, or simply chat on the phone. Because many of the volunteers at the American Cancer Society and the AMS Cancer Information and Counseling Line (CICL) are cancer survivors, I found that talking with them was most encouraging. Their objectivity and personal knowledge, learned through experiencing a situation similar to mine, were very helpful in my critical decision-making.

If you live alone, or if the people you live with are difficult to bare your heart to, then I pray for God to send you someone with whom you can honestly share your needs. I did not want to be alone too much, if at all, once treatments were underway. Alone is definitely harder than together. You will find much comfort in the companionship of friends, another person in the room, or someone on the other end of the phone. I did. And whenever I was tempted to withdraw, I decided it was healthiest to just get out. Shopping, working, or making some phone calls made me feel connected to the "real" world.

Once you have finally taken the courageous step of letting everyone in on your new science project, don't be surprised if some of your friends or family members subtly withdraw. I had this experience and it surprised me–until I discovered through talking with other cancer survivors that they had encountered the same thing. It is anyone's guess why some people react this way to the news of your breast cancer. Speculations range from fear and an unwillingness to face their own immortality to simply feeling awkward and not knowing what to say or how to help. Some people just slip into a state of shock and park there for a while. Those who are able and choose to be involved in your life during this time will forever be engraved in your heart.

If you are reading this book because you know someone with breast cancer, remember the verse from Proverbs 17:17, "A friend loves at all times and a *sister* is born for adversity" (original text reads *brother*).

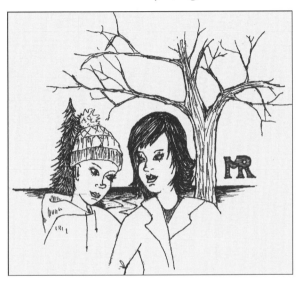

Today's Scripture

"Use hospitality one to another without grudging."
–I Peter 4:9 (KJV)

Quote

"Always do right–this will gratify some and astonish the rest."
–Mark Twain (1835-1910)

Prayer

Lord, in our weakened state, empower us
not to seek friends for ourselves,
but to find ways to give
some part of ourselves to another.
We rejoice in those friends you have encircled
around us and receive them as gifts from you.

May we cherish those friends we see daily
as well as those whose friendship
we long for. Thank you for exemplifying perfect
friendship by sharing Your life with us.
Amen

Musical Selection

Fantasia, Allemand, Gigue-From Bach Partita #3 in A Minor
—Johann Sebastian Bach (1685-1750)

Chapter 8
Kafka-esque Cancer

I found that when confronted with demoralizing, albeit life-preserving, medical procedures, there lurks the danger of assuming an attitude of infirmity or despair that disrupts faith-thoughts and threatens hope.

He fumbles at your spirit
As players at the keys
Before they drop full music on;
He stuns you by degrees,

Prepares your brittle substance
For the ethereal blow,
By fainter hammers, further heard,
Then nearer, then so slow

Your breath has time to straighten,
Your brain to bubble cool,—
Deals one imperial thunderbolt
That scalps your naked soul.

—Emily Dickinson

EVEN THOUGH I still didn't feel totally comfortable with radiation treatment, we scheduled an appointment with the radiation oncologist. I wanted to keep an open mind and learn the opinions of experts. After all, I was on a quest for cancer-free living. After giving me a very thorough examination the doctor told us that I was a good candidate for radiation since, aside from the cancer, I was in excellent health. He then left the room to review the films I had brought from various mammograms.

Dan and I were dismayed when, a few minutes later, the doctor returned to the room with the shocking news that he was not convinced that radiation would successfully treat the breast tissue. He had located another area on the mammogram films that he strongly suspected was cancer and recommended that I have another stereotactic biopsy to put his suspicion to the test. Now, stereotactic biopsies are not fun, but because I wanted to keep the healing process moving along and there was no other reasonable option, I agreed to it.

It was inconceivable to me then, as it is now, how the radiologists, the surgical oncologist, and all the others involved, had missed yet another area of cancer! Such is the elusive nature of cancer. If you have ever read a Franz Kafka novel, you will appreciate what this moment was like for me. I felt the sense of futility and frustrating tail-spinning that characterizes Kafka's writings. I had to read Kafka in college and the frustration of never arriving at a logical conclusion nearly drove me mad. And here it was again. I really felt I was locked in a Kafka novel, never to come to any conclusion at all.

We had chosen this particular radiation oncologist because he was one of the top experts in his field, and here he was telling us that he couldn't help us–at least not yet. Even though I had planned on chemotherapy and perhaps tamoxifen to follow, he strongly recommended another lumpectomy to remove more breast tissue. I'm not sure how we even managed to walk out of GBMC that morning. The doctor was kind, supportive, compassionate, professional, and we were sure he was telling us the truth. It's true: Sometimes the truth hurts. It hurt. Somehow we managed to find the car and drive home, stunned.

Ultimately, I would come to feel that this doctor had been instrumental in saving my life, as that still-loitering cancer might have spread and trespassed my health.

I had already read *Dr. Susan Love's Breast Book*, but I returned to it again, to search for answers. I read what I understood to mean that calcifications are precursors to breast cancer. I read that the greatest risk of getting breast cancer is *having had breast cancer*. Which meant it was very likely that I would someday have breast cancer on the left side. I wondered how much breast tissue would be left on the right side after that next lumpectomy. My surgeon told us he could reduce the left side to match the right side after I finished chemotherapy treatments. But I feared that cancerous cells exposed to the air might multiply faster, and that if any of the left breast tissue was *atypical hyperplasia*, this very well could happen. What if the calcifications in the left breast turned to cancer? What if they turned to cancer after I had already had a reduction surgery? What if there was cancer there *now*?

After all, areas of cancerous tissue had been missed before my meeting with the radiation oncologist. I was starting to feel that the breast cancer was like a ghost, showing up and then vanishing, and and then showing up again. I had to ask myself some difficult questions. How long did I want to deal with cancer and wonder if there was more about to crop up? Did I have the courage and the grace to be lopsided between surgeries and then live with the knowledge that I would need to watch both breasts closely for cancer developments? How long would I need to do this? Could I live the rest of my life this way? I had many questions—and very few answers. In spite of all the research that has been done, much more is needed for women to find answers to the questions they have in this crisis situation.

We pored over lots of medical references and talked over the risks of undetected cancer, and in the end Dan and I agreed about everything—although he left the final decision-making entirely up to me. The next morning I called my surgeon and told him I wanted a bilateral simple mastectomy. I wanted to get on with my life. He assured me that he and the radiation oncologist felt that they could probably still get it all. "Probably" was not a strong enough word for me at this point. My decision had been made; I wanted the bilateral mastectomy. It would take more than calculated, even scientific, speculation to reverse my decision.

Now the search for a reconstructive surgeon began. I knew that I wanted reconstruction immediately, even though many women choose to wait until after chemotherapy. Dan and I started asking our doctors and friends for names of good plastic surgeons. The one who was most highly recommended was not able to see me for three months. That wouldn't do. So I got his office to give me the name of another plastic surgeon, and we scheduled an office visit the following week.

I never realized how much I admired my own body until I was faced with losing it. But I found that when confronted with demoralizing, albeit life-preserving, medical procedures, there lurks the real danger of assuming an attitude of infirmity or despair that disrupts faith-thoughts and threatens hope. So you have to fend off this danger! How? By going on the offensive and meeting the thoughts of despair head-on, you can charge your belief system with hopeful attitudes. Speak words that affirm your divine citizenship and royalty will turn your thoughts to God's goodness. Speaking words that reveal your natural limitations will defeat despair. So choose your words carefully, for your soul will digest them recklessly!

Today's Scripture

"My soul melteth for heaviness; strengthen me according to Thy word."

–Psalm 119:28 (KJV)

Quote

"Success is to be measured not so much by the position that one has reached in life as by the obstacles which he has overcome."

–Booker T. Washington (1856-1915)

Prayer

Oh! God of all mercies, anchor my thoughts
in the surety of knowing that
because You are in control, there have been no
mistakes made that can harm me.
I seek Your face for wisdom, emboldened determination,
and fierceness with which to pursue
yet another phase of the cancer journey.
Grant me Your presence and may it consume me so

thoroughly that clarity of thought will direct my steps.

Amen

Musical selection

Poupee Valsante (Dancing Doll)

–Eduard Poldini (1869-1957

Chapter 9
The Haunted House

A Full Moon's Autumn Eve

A gentle breeze in my trees
Sound a soft, soothing welcome
As weary, I return from shopping.
On high above, the jostling leaves
Alone are moving on the oak–
They quietly wave an evening greeting!
Single clouds, dark blue and gray,
Edged all 'round in pearly white,
Float free, far beyond my counting!
Harvest's shy moon hides behind
A gauzy covering of palest gray–
'though earlier seen so broadly smiling!
And so–one last look above
Assures me God's still nearby
With scenes to set my heart rejoicing!

–Eugenia May Benner
(Poet and Author's Mother)

ALTHOUGH IT was not Halloween when Dan and I arrived at the plastic surgeon's office, the day would soon take a turn for the ghastly. The waiting room was crowded with people. And as I looked around, the atmosphere was decidedly gloomy. I looked on faces with no smiles, faces darkened with frustrated frowns. I saw people impatiently studying their watches, downcast eyes staring at the floor. The odor in the room was stale, heavy, and I felt as though I were gasping for breath. Well, I thought, at least the plastic surgeon was busy: He must be at least *fairly* good to have all these patients. Or, hmm, maybe he just accepts a lot of different insurance plans. As we waited uncomfortably for over forty minutes, my spirit plunged, while other spirits seemed to haunt us.

At long last my name was called, and my hopefulness quickly returned, because I earnestly believed I would find in this surgeon my miracle worker. We were escorted into a gray, sterile examination room where the doctor quickly and succinctly explained the tram flap and the tissue expander reconstruction options. I don't recall exactly what he said next, but he clearly conveyed to both Dan and me that he wasn't especially excited or optimistic about either option. "What other options are there?" we asked.

"None," he said. Dan was getting angry. We had hoped for respectful restoration and had met with derisive demolition.

Bewildered and confused, we asked to see pictures of previous patients who had undergone both types of reconstruction. (I had read somewhere to ask to see pictures.) The doctor reluctantly asked his assistant to bring in the photo album. I assure you that this was not the kind of album you would pass around at family gatherings or dinner parties–unless maybe it was Halloween. The pictures were horrible! Every one of them looked disfigured and ghastly scarred. Somehow I could not select any of them that I would want to look like.

Dan and I were starting to understand why this doctor was not too excited about reconstructive surgery. He wouldn't have time for another office visit, so he asked then and there if we had any further questions. Before we left, he told us to call him if we wanted to schedule something... We didn't. *Schedule what?* we wondered. A freak show?

We felt humiliated, angry, and betrayed as we left his office and ran for our car. It was not until that moment, just then, that I felt as though God had forsaken me. Had the previous months been nothing more than a really sick prank that had been pulled on us? "Happy Halloween," I blubbered to Dan, who rejoined sympathetically and pragmatically with, "We'll keep shopping."

After crying away the rest of that afternoon and night with a certifiable pity party, I woke up angry, wondering how many women would have a similar experience. I decided that when disfigurement becomes a prerequisite to health, your value system must be deeper than skin. I read Proverbs 13:12: "Hope deferred makes the heart sick, but when desire comes it is a tree of life." For the first time since I was diagnosed with breast cancer I understood the truth of this verse. I felt really sick and prayed for hope to find me quickly.

I had been to many motivational seminars, so I understood the connection between cause and effect. Believe me, I had a cause. A few days passed before the cause propelled us into action. Time was of the essence. The mastectomy surgery was already scheduled, and I was determined to have reconstruction at the same time as the mastectomies. I would need to find some wonderful surgeon to perform the task, and I had to find him or her fast!

We made numerous phone calls and searched the Web for God's response to the Halloween haunt. Then one day a woman who was a cancer survivor came to my office and asked to see me. She had heard that I had not found a plastic surgeon in whose hands I felt secure. She told me that she was delighted with the successful and beautiful reconstruction a local plastic surgeon had performed on her. She left me his name and number and made me promise to call him. She would call ahead and let the staff know the urgency of my situation. What a blessing!

As soon as I could clear my office, I picked up the phone and nervously called Dr. James Paskert. The secretary, Katy, was already expecting my call, and she delightfully answered my questions and scheduled an appointment for the very next day. What time was convenient for me?

The warm waiting room was not stuffed with bodies. The staff was friendly and did not appear flustered or harried. Dan and I were invited into a conference office where we viewed a video about reconstruction options. The doctor shared pictures of patients in the various stages of reconstruction. The final pictures looked good. I recognized them as breasts, well contoured and with minimal scarring. In several photographs, the post-cancer breasts actually looked better than the pre-cancer breasts! My sick and nervous stomach of the past week was starting to settle down as hopefulness took its rightful place in my heart. God's provisions are always timely. The surgical oncologist and the plastic surgeon were able to coordinate their schedules.

Now I braced for the imminent image change from which there would be no return.

I found the promise of Psalm 30:5 so true and comforting: "Weeping may endure for a night, but joy comes in the morning." In times of real or perceived danger we naturally arm ourselves with self-preservation—a strong God-given instinct. This appropriate response to a crisis is designed much like a temporary adrenalin rush to help us respond to a threat. When the provision replaces the problem, we can give self-preservation a rest. Because of the anxiety and intensity of our cancer battle, our runaway minds may continue to stampede the battlefield. When this occurs, God in His grace will recapture our thoughts and recall to our minds the premise of His character. We can safely lay down our weapons, while keeping the shield of faith securely strapped on.

Today's Scripture

"What then shall we say to these things? If God is for us, who can be against us?"

–Romans 8:31 (NKJV)

Quote

"Most people would rather die than think; in fact, they do so."

–Bertrand Russell (1872-1970)

Prayer

Father, thank You that when we are haunted by
our past, our illness, our self-image,
You are there to remind us that You are for us.
In loving ourselves, we will be free to love others.
May Your Holy Spirit quicken to our memories
eternal hope, faith, and above all, patience,
while we wait to see Your provisions.

Amen

Musical selection

Symphonie Concertante I: K.364
      –Wolfgang Amadeus Mozart (1756-1791)

Chapter 10
Finding the Purpose

I began to feel that I was not suffering at all. The cup of life had simply passed my way, and I would take a drink.

Faith, mighty faith, the promise sees,
And looks to that alone;
Laughs at life's impossibilities,
And cries, It shall be done!

–From "Hymn No. 360"
Charles Wesley (1707-1788)

THE CULTURE of the high school Dan and I serve promotes intimate friendships between students and staff. When the student body learned that I had breast cancer, their response was one of stunned disbelief. Susan, our high school guidance counselor, suggested that I speak to the senior class about my breast cancer situation. "They have questions," she said. "They're upset about it."

Okay. What was I going to tell these students–that God is not faithful after all?

Although many weeks had passed since my diagnosis, I was just starting to believe the news myself! I had not yet sought out the purpose of my cancer in His plan. I had been scrambling to get to doctor appointments. I was simply putting one foot in front of the other, while the promise of Romans 8:28 that "all things work together for good" lurked coyly in the back of my mind.

I had only about an hour before I would stand before the students. I went into my office and closed the door and my mind and pried open my heart to look inside. I found some anger. It was not directed at God;

it was just wholesome anger. I pondered on why I wasn't directing my anger toward God, for He seemed to be the only one I could truly point a finger at. My mind turned towards the suffering of others in our world. I pictured veterans with no limbs, students paralyzed from birth or from an accident. I thought about an applicant at our school whose face and head had been severely burned in a fire; skin grafts had not done much to restore her beauty. She had only a few shafts of hair left, growing sporadically. Her mother lovingly applied bows of pastel colors to make her feel pretty. I thought of Vanessa who had contracted a rare eye disease and by the age of twelve could not recall how many corrective surgeries she'd undergone–which had failed to *correct* her vision. And then there were Roseanne and Donna–beautiful, godly women of faith– who had died so unfairly from breast cancer.

I thought of the little old lady who lives on our street. She's just adorable as she walks her dog in an old-fashioned, apron-style housecoat. She moves so slowly and we sense her suffering when we drive past and catch a glimpse of her. My heart began to ache for suffering children; some in our community whose personalities will be forever scarred by the abuse and violence in their worlds. Orphans in Romania and in India, in Africa, Afghanistan, and Iraq. Children everywhere left helpless and hopeless. In my heart I prayed for these dear ones, prayed Psalm 27:10: "When my father and mother forsake me, the LORD will take me up." The suffering in the world is so enormous, and my suffering was so small in contrast.

I began to feel that I was not suffering at all. The cup of life had simply passed my way, and I would take a drink. Life's complex patterns of dark and light, of sorrow and joy, can only be measured against eternity. With confidence in my God's compassion and loyalty to the human race, I felt sure that He would carry me through. I considered the *unexplainableness* of God's mercies to comfort us in our weakness and suffering and how it could be that we feel His presence closer to us in illness. Why do we feel him so closely, His comfort permeating our pain and fear?

I discovered that God is the Master of the art of turning a curse into a blessing and that the secret to inner peace and joy is to look for the blessings. They are always there, although at times they come wrapped in mysterious disguises that only the careful and thoughtful observer can see through.

My secretary knocked on my office door. "The senior class is gathering. Are you still going over to speak with them?" Yes, I was, and as I stood before them I saw that their faces were white, somber, and scared. The stark silence in the room hovered above the assembly like a dark rain cloud. I could sense the students' love and compassion, mingled with sorrow and fear. Before long, the eternal question "Why?" posed itself.

The answer was now clear.

Why *not*? Why not *me*? What is so special about me that I should not suffer while the world is suffering? True, I am God's child with special privileges, and one of those privileges is that I can identify with others through suffering. Would I choose this for myself? *Ha!* Certainly not. But since one of life's most terrifying challenges had chosen me, I chose to think of God's words of comfort, healing, and abiding presence–chose to *ponder* them, to make them the center of my conscious thought life. Soon I could *feel* His arms underneath me, His spirit propelling me forward with a sense of security and fervency that I could only explain as supernatural. I began to understand that suffering would do two things: extract patience and magnify grace.

When the assembly was over, the students' faces looked relieved and revitalized. Many of them approached me to offer words of encouragement and promises of prayer. My mission was successful, as I had wanted them to feel God's goodness in the midst of all our fear and apprehension.

But what about those days when the shadow of unbelief haunts our confidence? The dark shadows of unbelief may come wrapped up as a bad mood, as physical exhaustion, or as piercing pain. At these junctures of disgruntlement, I find it best to quiet my mind and my mouth, drink some ginger tea, and wait on God to restore my soul. The blessing of feeling Him near us may not be constant, but simply analyzing our faith is surely an exercise in futility. God has planned around our moments of unbelief. His plan includes our vulnerability and His guarantee is true: "He who calls you is faithful, who also will do it" (I Thessalonians 5:24).

Today's Scripture

"He is despised and rejected by men, a Man of sorrows and acquainted with grief. And we hid, as it were, our faces from Him: He was despised and we did not esteem Him."

–Isaiah 53:3 (NKJV)

Quote

"O divine Master, grant that I may not so much seek to be consoled as to console; to be understood as to understand; to be loved as to love. For it is in giving that we receive; it is in pardoning that we are pardoned; and it is in dying that we are born to eternal life."

–St. Francis of Assisi, *The Peace Prayer*

Prayer

Lord, keep me from distress, defeat, distraction, and dismay.
As I look up to heaven, let me delightfully embrace
the joy of encouraging and loving others.
Amen

Musical Selection

Concerto No. 2

–Sergei Rachmaninoff (1873-1943)

Chapter 11
Mastectomies Double-Take

The silence and the vast, open heavens, still and yet
powerful, spoke to me of God's majesty and dominion
and therein my soul found the rest it needed, preparing
for a surgery that seemed so far from nature,
and yet so much a part of God's provision.

IT WAS LATE October and the autumn leaves of Maryland had peaked in their brilliant colors. The air was crisp, but occasional warm days whispered promises of summers yet to come. All my autumn icons were in place: the harvest wreaths on the front double doors; the hay-stuffed wooden crate full of tumbling gourds at the corner of the entry way; the scarecrows with their happy faces; the jack-o'-lantern cast a warm glow on evenings not too cold for us to swing on the deck.

This is the bittersweet time of year. The crunch of leaves beneath my feet draws out the earnest vigor of the schoolhouse child in me. Yet knowing the bitter cold that will follow, I brace myself for the coming winter months when I will extract less from the great outdoors and more from indoor projects. The smell of the grass after the last mow of the season propels me into charting our winter course–the traditional distractions that keep our family patient and occupied as we await a new spring. There was always our daughter Karissa's birthday celebration, the Susquehanna Symphony Orchestra concerts, Thanksgiving and Christmas festivities, trips to New York and local theater.

The autumn after my diagnosis demanded a different course, a course that included the double mastectomies scheduled for October 30. On the evening of October 29, I lay out in the yard on my back staring at the brilliant stars twinking in the clear sky. Dan and our children,

Daniel and Karissa, joined me. As we lay on the ground feeling the cool dampness of dew, the dazzling stars seemed to smile promises of hope on me. The silence and the vast, open heavens, still and yet so powerful, spoke to me of God's majesty and dominion and therein my soul found the rest it needed to prepare for a surgery that seemed so far from nature, and yet so much a part of God's provision.

Proverbs 20:24, 27 says, "Man's goings are of the LORD: how can a man then understand his way? ... The spirit of man is the candle of the LORD, searching all the inward parts of the soul." It was enough for me to know that God knew my way, so I trusted that the hard decisions I had made would all work out for the best. I surrendered my worries to God's caring nature and found peace of body and mind.

By 9:00 P.M. my resolve was firm. I focused on the morning's plan and prepared for action, and, declaring myself a vehement, victimless, knee-knocking *victor*, I left the night air behind. I rehearsed a mental list of mastectomy and reconstruction benefits to steady my nerves:

1   My post-cancer recurrence rate would drop to two percent once the surgery and the chemotherapy were complete.
2   My bazooms would be a perfect, perky match, making me look younger–a great incentive at forty-five years old!
3   "Best Breasts" was doing the plastic surgery; rumor had it that Dr. Paskert's colleagues amiably gave him this nickname for his plastic surgery craftsmanship.

I mused over Philippians 4:6-7, which says, "Be anxious for nothing, but in everything by prayer and supplication with thanksgiving, let your requests be made known unto God. And the peace of God, which passes all understanding, shall keep your hearts and minds through Christ Jesus."

God had heard my prayers, supplications, and requests, and I was enjoying the benefit of having my mind "kept." Dan and I turned in and slept soundly until the alarm rang early to announce the start of a day that was set apart for a unique purpose. It was still dark outside as we drove to GBMC. We rolled down the windows and let the cool air rush in and held hands in the silence, certain that my life and health were in God's hands.

I remained calm throughout the surgical preparation process, although we had a bit of a delay waiting for an operating room to become available after an emergency surgery. As we waited in the cubicle, I was decked in my enchanting hospital surgery outfit, complete with rubber-soled socks and blue elastic trimmed hat.

Forty minutes passed, and I was just beginning to grow a bit impatient when the deafening noise of a power saw began. I was horror-struck; the clamor was coming from the cubicle right next to mine. Now let's be real, here... I was just about to have both my breasts cut out, and the power saw was becoming louder.

Would you be laughing at the irony or screaming at the madness? No amount of spiritual exercise could have prepared me for this one! I approached the nurses' station and, with diplomatic composure, I inquired about the commotion, knowing all the while that God had to have scheduled such an ironic situation. At least I chose to see Him looking down at me and chuckling!

The nurses politely explained that the noise was indeed a power saw. The person in that cubicle was having a cast removed. "Could they please stop until I go in for my surgery?" I asked. "No, they cannot stop in the middle of removing the cast," the nurse replied, sympathetically. I muttered some comment about "psychological harassment," to which the nurses responded by quickly relocating us to a room in another hallway with a door that closed.

Fortunately, Dr. Paskert arrived shortly thereafter, saying he was ready for me. His easygoing, tranquil manner made my short walk to the operating room easier. I lay down on the surgical stretcher, greeted my surgeons and nurses, joked a bit with the anesthesiologists who seem to be always equipped with a fresh batch of comic relief quips, and dozed off with a prayer.

The Angel

I dreamt a dream! What can it mean?
And that I was a maiden Queen
Guarded by an Angel mild:
Witless woe was ne'er beguiled!

And I wept both night and day,
And he wiped my tears away;
And I wept both day and night,
And hid from him my heart's delight.

So he took his wings, and fled;
Then the morn blushed rosy red.
I dried my tears, and armed my fears
With ten-thousand shields and spears.

Soon my Angel came again;
I was armed, he came in vain;
For the time of youth was fled,
And grey hairs were on my head.

–William Blake (1757-1827)

Today's Scripture

"Your two breasts *are* like two fawns, Twins of a gazelle, which feed among the lilies."

–Song of Solomon 4:5 (NKJV)

Quote

"I've had a wonderful time, but this wasn't it."

–Groucho Marx (1895-1977)

Prayer

Lord, I offer to you my diseased breasts
on the altar of healing. May the surgeons
work well together as one removes
the old and the other begins the new.
Thank you for the gift of reconstruction.

I am amazed at how relaxed and relieved I feel–
I rejoice in Your presence, knowing You will guide
my surgeons' hands…
while "Fly Me to the Moon"
plays on the radio in the background!
A Glorious AMEN!

Musical Selection

Our 1 D Tafelmusik Ii
–George Philipp Telemann (1681-1767)

Chapter 12
Recovery

Allowing God to work on areas of our lives in which we desire growth or change will lead to improved clarity of thought and purpose.

I HEARD DAN'S voice and saw his shadow in the room. His hand was resting gently on my arm, from which poked all sorts of tubes. Minimal pain is what I had expected; maximum pain was what I felt. The room looked hazy and gray, and that groggy, post-anesthesia hangover had me feeling sick. For all my groaning, I could barely open my eyes. As soon as my eyelids were light enough to open, a nurse injected something into one of my thighs and, just like that, I was sleeping again.

The day passed into night. I asked Dan to stay, because I couldn't so much as pull up a blanket or shift my body for myself. He found a comfortable chair, pillow, and blanket and waited on me throughout the night. Sometime the next morning the nurses helped me into a chair. I was very dizzy from morphine and pain, and started to dry-heave uncontrollably.

The medication was soon changed to something lighter, and I began to think clearly, although the pain was still excruciating. I exhorted myself to get my act together, to separate pain from promise. I fought mentally to move the past into the present and focused on my goal of getting home. I kept recalling Psalm 39:4, "Lord, make me know mine end, and the measure of my days, what it is; that I may know how frail I am."

I was very frail, but within three days I was at home, with visiting nurses scheduled to check in periodically to tend to my drains and chart my progress toward recovery.

I needed pain management during the days following surgery. The pain medication helped, to an extent, but I did not want to depend solely on that. I tried physical therapy for the first few days, along with massage therapy. I was fortunate enough to find a massage therapist, Eric Wilson, whose primary interest in helping to alleviate suffering inspired him to reduce his fees for post-surgery clients. Eric's massage therapy practice is under contract to provide therapeutic massage to patients at Upper Chesapeake Medical Center and Harford Memorial Hospital. These hospitals offer massage therapy to help manage pain and facilitate healing. Eric has volunteered many hours at these health care facilities to help develop their massage therapy programs, and he also trains volunteers in Nurturing Touch, a service provided to patients free of charge.

I went for massage therapy daily for a while, then three times a week, then weekly. And I credit much of my healing during that time to his hands, which were an extension of God's touch.

The expanders had been inserted during the mastectomy procedure. Expanders are the empty post-surgical breast pouches that are inserted with the objective of expanding them gradually with saline to stretch the skin to prepare it for permanent breast implants. With the expanders in place, I was now ready to begin the process of reconstruction.

Every week or so, Dr. Paskert inserted more saline in the expander pouch through a valve that is located with a magnet. When the skin is expanded, it can be rather uncomfortable, so it is done slowly over a period of time. Once the desired cup size is achieved, several weeks must pass before the expander, which is temporary, can be removed and replaced by the permanent implant. At long last, the results are marvelous, and I am delighted with my beautifully contoured shape. As Dr. Paskert says, they are not divine creations, but God "looks over our shoulders" as we co-create, restoring beauty to the broken vessel.

I feel compelled to mention that if you feel you do not have a reasonably strong tolerance for pain, you may want to consider waiting a while before beginning reconstruction by expanders. With each injection of additional saline, the skin expands, and because the expanders are placed in a fresh mastectomy wound, it can be extremely painful. This is true for the first six to eight weeks of the recovery period, but the pain is especially excruciating during the first week. I do not regret having chosen to proceed as I did, but your personal level of comfort is something to consider when making this decision.

The scars do take a while to heal and this presents another test of patience. But in the meantime, they serve as a reminder that each new day is a gift of grace. Fairly new on the market at the time of this writing are the scar therapy cosmetic pads that speed along the scar-fading process. If your doctor agrees that they are safe for you to use, I highly recommend them, as they were very effective for me.

The season of breast cancer struggle can last for a while as you progress through the healing process. It may be a good year and half, or perhaps even two or more years, depending on your treatments, before you feel that you are back to a normal routine, sleeping soundly, and not turning your thoughts toward cancer daily.

A big part of the healing process includes the healing of the mind and heart as well as the body. Reflecting more frequently on God's gift of life may find you exploring your past, learning from experiences which, perhaps, you had not slowed down long enough to consider deeply. Allowing God to work on areas of our lives in which we desire growth or change leads to improved clarity of thought and purpose. Self-acceptance, forgiveness, resentment, fear, sadness, and anger may all be part of God's transforming process for you. Releasing past hurts to God will allow you to heal more freely and fully.

Blessed Breast Cancer Be-Attitudes

Blessed are those who focus on solutions and provisions, when they have more problems than most. *Be* thankful you have the chance to heal.

Blessed are those who love themselves as God does, even when they feel unlovely. *Be* available to receive His love.

Blessed are those who rejoice in each new day, who recognize the magic of a breeze and a sunset. *Be* true to yourself and do the things that you enjoy.

Blessed are those who cry when their hair falls out, but have fun with fashionable wigs. *Be* quick to see the humor in ridiculous situations.

Blessed are those who find His grace sufficient, defying doubt, discouragement, and despair. *Be* looking for the blessing.

Blessed are those who are not able to endure; for He will carry them. *Be* okay with your own limitations.

Blessed are those who mourn; for they shall be comforted. Indeed. *Be* reassured that joy comes in the morning.

Today's Scripture

"I drew them with gentle cords, with bands of love, and I was to them as those who take the yoke from their neck. I stooped and fed them."

–Hosea 11:4 (NKJV)

Quote

"Have a heart that never hardens, and a temper that never tires, and a touch that never hurts."

–Charles Dickens (1812-1870)

Prayer

Lord, let not my heart be hardened by pain
and weariness of the way. Let me not tire
of Your temperament of peace,
and may I understand in a deeper way

the need for a loving touch.
Grant me life and healing so that
by some miracle of grace I might
touch someone with Your heart of love.
Amen

Musical Selection

Concertante in Eb Flute, Clarinet, Violin Op. 70
–Franz Kromer (1759-1831)

Massage & the Healing Connection

By Eric Wilson, C.M.T., N.C.T.M.B.

PROPER MASSAGE techniques may be beneficial to cancer patients. Touch may help prevent tumor proliferation as it reduces the body's stress levels. High levels of these substances have been linked to tumor growth.

You should choose a massage therapist who is licensed in his or her state and holds the credential of national certification. Also, the massage therapist should have experience working with people with cancer. The benefits of pain minimization, stress reduction, and compassionate touch through the hands of a qualified massage therapist will have a lasting effect on the emotional, mental, and physical condition of the cancer patient.

Eric Wilson is a board certified massage therapist and president of Applied Massage Therapy of Harford County (Maryland), Inc., which specializes in pain management and stress reduction. Eric volunteers with the National Certification Board of Therapeutic Massage and Bodywork on the eligibility review panel, and he sits on the Massage Therapy Advisory Committee to the Maryland Board of Chiropractic Examiners.

Chapter 13
Thanksgiving Approaches

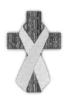

The sadness of some memories is mixed with other,
beautiful memories of people who loved and cried
and cared for me during those long months.
Perhaps they will remain with me forever, a symbol
of both human suffering and human compassion.

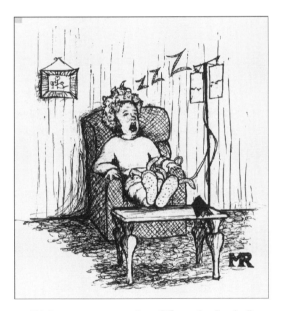

"A heart at peace gives life to the body."
–Proverbs 14:30 (NKJV)

I RECALL TRYING to eat heartily at Thanksgiving, as I imagined it might be the last time I would enjoy food for a while, although in general my appetite had decreased. I was scheduled to begin adjuvant chemotherapy treatments on November 29. Since the tumor was larger than originally thought (over one centimeter) and was poorly differentiated, Dr. Chaudhry recommended that I receive four chemotherapy cycles of Cytoxin and Adriamycin.

Dan and I had met a few times with Dr. Madhu Chaudhry at GBMC, and we found her to be helpful in educating us about research results on cases like mine. She was at once reassuring that I could get through the chemotherapy treatments and warmly sympathetic about the challenges of the treatment. I had been tentative about chemotherapy, but Dan persuaded me to go ahead with the treatment because the risks of side-effects were far less than the risks of non-treatment in my case.

Much to my surprise, the morning of November 29 was far more challenging for me than the morning of October 30, when we had headed out for the bilateral mastectomy. I was fearful that morning as I got in the car and Dan drove us to GBMC once again. Though the office and nursing staff were very supportive, there was a dense sadness in the air as I looked around at some other patients who had already lost their hair. Some patients seemed relaxed with the routine, while others looked as if they thought they were going to die at any moment.

The first treatment seemed easy. My veins were good, so there was no fussing with getting the meds hooked up. The staff explained to us in detail about the drugs I would receive and their possible side-effects. One thing was clear: With this combination of medications I would *definitely* lose my hair.

The time passed quickly, and in about three hours Dan and I were headed for home. I felt fine; I wanted to go shopping just to prove that I was fine, but Dan nixed that idea. A short while after arriving home, I started to feel a bit strange, and by 7:00 P.M. I had the worst headache imaginable and was vomiting over and over again. Oh my, so *this* is chemotherapy.

I recall admitting to myself then that I was sick. Was something really wrong? Was this a normal response? I called Dr. Chaudhry who asked me a number of questions and advised me to take various medications that she had prescribed and that I had on-hand. Eventually, I went to sleep, curled up tight and, even under my down comforter, still cold.

I smiled, remembering that a third grade student had come into my office one day declaring that the medication the doctor had given him had made his stomach sick, and he was now feeling rather "obnoxious"! The word he was apparently looking for was "nauseous." Well, chemotherapy made me obnoxiously nauseous, but the good news is that within a few days, the nausea subsided, and I was back on track.

I learned to psych myself out by pretending that I had the flu. It helped me to be patient with the sickish feeling, and to remember that within a few days I would feel much better. Subsequent treatments were not as bad, and good communication with Dr. Chaudhry resulted in more effective anti-nausea and headache medications.

As predicted, about two weeks later my hair started to fall out. Karissa and I went to the wig salon where they gave me a chic short haircut. But within just a few more days, I could see there was no point in trying to preserve the hair, so I put my head over the bathroom sink and shaved it all off. I recall pretending that I was about to play a major role in a new hit movie that required me to present myself bald! *Ha!* I thought of people who choose to wear a shaved head, although I had to admit that most of the people I could think of were, alas, men!

Thankfully (and mercifully), I had a beautiful wig which I had bought weeks previously, as I knew for sure that I would not care for the bald look after all. But then again, you never know until you try it. The weather was cold and when I was at home I constantly wore a soft, black Columbia ski hat that I borrowed from my son, Daniel. It looked great with big hoop earrings and was really warm.

The hat, along with the wigs and other reminders of my battle in the ring with cancer, are now folded and neatly packed away in a drawer not used for any other purpose. I often wonder why I keep them and when I will have the courage to throw them away. The sadness of some memories is mixed with other, beautiful memories of people who loved and cried and cared for me during those long months. Perhaps they will remain with me forever, a symbol of both human suffering and human compassion.

Chemotherapy is to healing what labor pains are to childbirth. The dreadful anticipation is far worse than the actual event. Nevertheless, I found chemotherapy to be the most difficult part of the cancer treatment. People were compassionate, and for that I was grateful. The weakness of my body invited me to sympathize too much with myself, and I had to resist self-pity, while being realistic with my need for rest. I must admit to times when, although my body was in the Lois Harvey Infusion Center, my mind was in the critical care mental health unit. It was in turning self-pity into self-love by receiving God's embrace that enabled me to move powerfully into the next phase of healing.

Chemotherapy Tips

1. Drink lots of water right before an infusion. It may help the nurse to locate your veins more easily.

2. Drink lots of water after an infusion, as it helps to flush the chemo out quickly. Since it does its job immediately, there's no need for it to linger in your system.

3. Iced peppermint tea with honey can help with nausea. I brought a 12-ounce bottle of my home-made iced brew with me to each treatment and sipped on it throughout the duration.

4. Consider a portacath if you will require long-term treatment. Your surgeon and medical oncologist can discuss the advantages with you, so you can make a decision best suited for you. If you don't use a portacath, then exercise your arms on the way to chemotherapy. Raising your arms over your head, or simply extending them out and up, will help get the blood flowing more strongly and may make venous access easier.

5. Avoid hot beverages, especially during treatment and for a week following treatment. The heat may encourage mouth

sores. In the event that you do get a mouth sore, notify your oncologist at once, as proper medication will clear it up promptly.

6. Keep some crackers on your nightstand. Eating even one cracker about 10 minutes before getting out of bed can help with morning nausea.

7. If smells bother you, and they will, communicate with your family or those you live with. On chemo days and up to three days later, my family knew that cooking was off-limits. The smells alone would be enough to make me nauseous, so they would order in sandwiches, make salads, or eat something cold. Even with these precautions, I usually stayed in bed with the blankets over my head until the food was cleared out of the way.

8. When you do feel like eating, eat! Chemotherapy is a bit like pregnancy in that you may crave something strange and just need to eat it. My doctor advised me not to ignore the cravings; probably there was some nutrient my body needed that was associated with the craving. I rarely eat pizza or hamburgers, but for some reason, on chemo-recovery days, these were strong cravings. My oncologist explained that it was the fat in those things that I was actually craving. So go ahead and indulge, just don't get carried away, or the extra pounds will carry you away!

9. Keep frozen treats around, such as Popsicles and Italian ice.

10. Avoid caffeine, tomatoes, green peppers, onions, and garlic before and after chemotherapy, as they can cause acid in the stomach and add to the nausea concern.

11. Keep your distance from anyone who may have a cold or the flu, since your immune system will be weakened during this time.

12. Avoid hand-shaking as that is a sure way to pick up un-friendly germs. If you become ill with the common cold or the flu, it may mean postponing chemotherapy treatments.

13. If you cannot or choose not to transport yourself to and from chemotherapy sessions, several of the cancer groups will help you by finding transportation. Specifically, Road to Recovery, sponsored by the American Cancer Society, provides volunteer drivers who will drive you not only to chemotherapy appointments, but to your other dozens of appointments as well!

Today's Scripture

"A Psalm of Thanksgiving. Make a joyful shout to the Lord, all you lands!"

–Psalm 100:1 (NKJV)

Quote

"If there is no struggle, there is no progress."

–Frederick Douglas (1818-1895)

Prayer

Heavenly Father, I thank You for giving us
the divine power to choose Your thoughts
of healing, goodness, and strength
over our own thoughts of fear, dread,
anxiety,and helplessness.
Thank You for carrying us
as we put one foot in front of the other,
offering thanks and praise with our mouths…
sometimes by blind faith.
Amen

Musical Selection

Symphony #26 in D Minor-Lamentatione
–Franz Joseph Haydn (1732-1809)

Chapter 14
Dodging Dark & Dismal Days

I recognized their staring eyes right away, for they had been mine in my pre-cancer days. Like the rest of the world, I never wanted to suffer.

THE MONTHS passed slowly after that first mention of cancer. It seemed our lives were somehow engulfed in a huge capsule, a bubble floating around in the real world, but not truly a part of it. The countless trips to doctors' offices, hospitals, labs, and the Lois Harvey Infusion Center never became *routine*, and Dan and I never fully embraced them. We kept our arms around each other mostly, and maybe that's why the bubble did not burst.

When we are well, most of us yearn for vacation time, but what we thirst for when our bodies are restricted or confined through illness is our *normal routine*. I could feel the pulse of God pushing me to resist despondency and dullness of spirit, and I found many distractions to get me through those less than pleasant months of working toward wellness. Dan stayed busy distracting me when long days at home became mundane.

There were simple trips to Dunkin' Donuts for frozen drinks, followed by long drives on country roads. Board games and cards became hilarious, especially when I was on pain-killers and I couldn't distinguish the rules of Hearts from the rules of Spades; needless to say, I was not winning any hands. We threw our own Super Bowl party and, to my astonishment, when I ate some chicken wings, they stayed down. From furniture shopping to wallpapering, Dan's creative genius was always at work.

Alas, my hair was no more. One Saturday I could not stand to wear that wig another minute, yet I just had to get out of the house, to go anywhere—to just get out! Dan's idea this time was to travel to a remote mall where I was sure I wouldn't see anyone I knew. I wore a turban, and we ate Mexican food. Now, some women look absolutely stunning in a turban. I am not one of them. I look shrunken and ill in a turban. Our excursion that Saturday turned out to be an important experience for me, because it was the first time I was aware that people were staring at me. They were not staring through eyes of mockery, shock, or pity, but through eyes that said, "My God, I hope that is never me!"

I recognized their staring eyes right away, for they had been mine in my pre-cancer days. Like the rest of the world, I never wanted to suffer.

The best of all possible distractions is an experience that fills the soul with all good things! And there is nothing quite like church fellowship to enliven the spirit as you rejoice in truth and hear God's Word proclaimed. Unfortunately, though, many times I was simply too sick to make it to church on account of chemotherapy or some post-surgical condition. Often Dan would stay home with me to ward off the daunting doldrums of solitude. Solitude has its own divine essence, but I did not find it aromatic during cancer days. Many times we would call the church and ask Jeannie, our church receptionist, to put us on a speaker phone so we could listen to the church service.

Now Jeannie is someone I wish you could meet. She is an incredible woman of faith who was stricken with Multiple Sclerosis years ago. Jeannie's acceptance of her MS reflects her bold trust in God's divine plan for her. Her compassion toward others is so heart-felt that I must believe that she doesn't own a mirror, for she never looks at herself, though she is lovely to behold. So just hearing Jeannie's voice on the other end of the phone was enough to brighten my day. Her beautiful attitude of grace reflects her inner elegance and self-esteem. She is one terrific dismal day dodger!

Seek out the Jeannies in your life, whose joy is contagious.

Another way to dodge a dismal day is to get busy doing something for someone else. If you are lonely, consider picking up the phone to cheer up another cancer patient you may have met during treatment.

Other things I found helpful in dodging dismal days included: cleaning closets, cleaning desk drawers, arranging flowers, and planning for Christmas. Sewing, walking, gardening, music, board games, and romantic movies all worked for me. I watched all my old favorite movies during the dismal days. In case you're interested the list included *An Affair to Remember, You've Got Mail, Groundhog Day, Miracle on 34th Street, Sabrina,* and *Sleepless in Seattle.* I truly could not bear violence or conflicts of any kind during the cancer ordeal, so happy-sappy movies were big hits in the Baker's theater!

The best dismal day dodgers of all, though, were my children Karissa and Daniel, who brought me great gladness and comfort. Their presence brought to life the truth of the verse, "Blessed be the LORD, who daily loads us with benefits, even the God of our salvation" (Psalm 68:19). Open our eyes, Lord, that we may not miss daily blessings and that we might experience the refreshing of our souls, dodging dismal days as we make the most of our natural and supernatural resources.

Sylvia's Breast Cancer Amplified Version of Ecclesiastes 3:1-8

To everything there is a season;
will I see another summer?

And a time to every purpose under heaven;
this purpose I cannot grasp.

A time to be born and a time to die;
will it be soon?

A time to plant *seeds of hope*;
and a time to pluck up *unforgiveness.*

A time to kill the cancer,
and a time to heal me!

A time to break down *and cry*, and a time to laugh
when your wig falls off in the wind!

A time to mourn *those who lose the battle*,
and a time to dance–
on the last chemo treatment day!

A time to cast away stones;
people in glass houses shouldn't throw them!

A time to gather stones together
to build relationships, new and old.

A time to embrace *everyone you see,*
we all need hugs.

A time to refrain from embracing–
during chemo so you won't catch germs!

A time to get *flowers and cards,*
And a time to lose *hopefully not everything you eat,*
but a few pounds will do.

A time to keep *treasured memories of those you love.*

A time to cast away *hostility and anger.*

A time to rend *my hair out if I had any.*

A time to sew *new clothes for*
the many shapes of reconstruction.

A time to keep silence *because God is in heaven,*
And a time to speak *of His new mercies.*

A time to love *everyone–*
you never know what someone is going through.

A time to hate *the cancer and fight back.*
A time of war *within my body;*
A time of peace *within my soul.*

Today's Scripture

"Thou wilt shew me the path of life; in thy presence is fullness of joy; at thy right hand there are pleasures for evermore."

–Psalm 16:11(KJV)

Quote

"...Ice pellets gently sprinkled with snow dollops on evergreens...some mounded as igloos of white sugar as a pure, fleece blanket. Let me never forget that this is my Father's world."

–Gail Kunkel (writer and author's friend)

Prayer

Thank You my Father, for the pleasures
small and great that we discover along the way.
The surprise of beauty and the wonder of creativity–
I marvel at it all! Thank You for sunrises and sunsets,
buds and blossoms, caterpillars and butterflies–
You truly are quite a creative genius.
Much love, Your daughter, Sylvia

Musical Selection

Franzosische Overture in B Minor BWV831
–Johann Sebastian Bach (1685-1750)

Chapter 15
Trial Blessings

> *The value of life is clearer now. The sun's glow is warmer, the*
> *river more serene, even the bird's song is celebrated.*

Time is passing
as the river ripples gently along,
The rising sun excites life as
I arise to hear the morning song.
Today's vigor resigns in contentment
that feels like a porch in summer.
Tomorrow's path is calling me
to scout through new paths,
And know the joy of skipping along
to time passing.

Treasured trial blessings came in two phases for me. The first phase, the *Graced Out Phase*, got me through all the ugly stuff, the hassles, and the overwhelming sense of sudden tragedy. Consider Proverbs 27:7, which whets the appetite for God's love and mercy and delights our spiritual taste buds: "The full soul loathes an honeycomb; but to the hungry soul, every bitter thing is sweet."

During the *Graced Out Phase*, the famous poem "Footprints in the Sand" comes to mind. You might recall that the author observed that throughout her life journey there were always two sets of footprints, *except* during the lowest and saddest times in her life. Feeling deserted by God, the poet tells the Lord, "I don't understand why you left my side when I needed you most." To which the Lord replies that during those times of trial He had not deserted the sufferer but rather carried her in His arms to get her safely through. The one set of footprints was the

Lord's. Mysteriously, we are carried through the hardest times, and we know not how except to say that God is faithful. We sense God's caring arms beneath us and are confident that we shall not fall except into His care.

The second phase of blessings was the *Trial Aftermath Phase* that began slowly and gained momentum, never ceasing. In *Trial Aftermath* the reality of having been in the fire and coming out smelling like lavender rather than smoke brings with it a certain gusto for life that accentuates the positive in everything. A sense of power, clarity of direction, an insatiable appetite for life, the willingness to take risks when needed, the determination to pursue your dreams, are all a part of *Trial Aftermath*. In pre-cancer I knew everything about God by faith, but in post-cancer I was like John in the book of *Revelation*, all excited about having seen the glories of heaven! We cancer survivors, like others who have suffered, have truly tasted God's goodness and seen His glory; we have learned that He is faithful. Nothing is too hard for God. We know from personal experience that God is faithful in the worst trial, and that it is His faithfulness that takes the worry and apprehension out of life.

I have heard people say that getting cancer was a gift. I can only assume they mean that prior to the experience of cancer, they understood God's faithfulness only in theory. Now they understand it personally. If you lived a reserved life before cancer, you're likely to live abundantly once your treatment is over. You know that God will never leave you nor forsake you, so what's to fear?

Charge headlong into life and discover more of God's divine design for you. If you've not explored your own heart's desires, then take this down-time for some healthy self-reflection. With whom do you want to spend your time? For your time is a precious commodity. What hobbies are your passion or pleasure? Are you pursuing them?

If you are still in treatment, a great exercise on a dull day is to make notes of your vision for your life. Where do you see yourself in six months? In one year? In five years? Whom do you hope to influence? Whom do you want to help through this life? Develop a self-portrait through His eyes of grace. Do you enjoy quiet, peaceful settings or the bustle of city life? Maybe you love both. Do you want to paint? Sing? Swing? What is most important to you? Hopefully you will reflect God's honor back to Him through your life, as He has honored you with His. The value of life is clearer now. The sun's glow is warmer, the river more serene, even the bird's song is celebrated. With treatments coming to a close, we cherish each dawn as a priceless gift. Embrace each day fully and it will give back to you the kiss of God.

Life

Life, believe is not a dream
so dark as sages say;
Oft a little morning rain
foretells a pleasant day.

Sometimes there are clouds of gloom,
but these transient all;
If the shower will make the roses bloom,
O why lament its fall?

Rapidly, merrily,
life's sunny hours flit by,
Gratefully, cheerily
enjoy them as they fly!

What Death at times steps in,
and calls our Best away?
What though sorrow seems to win,
o'er hope, a heavy sway?

Yet hope again elastic springs,
unconquered, though she fell;
Still buoyant are her golden wings,
still strong to bear us well.

Manfully, fearlessly, the day of trial bear,
For gloriously, victoriously,
can courage quell despair!

–Charlotte Bronte (1817-1855)

Today's Scripture

"What then shall we say to these things? If God is for us, who can be against us?"

—Romans 8:31 (NKJV)

Quote

"But at my back I always hear Time's winged Chariot hurrying near."

—Andrew Marvel (1621-1678), "To His Coy Mistress"

Prayer

Cause me to give pause to the pace of this race
long enough to see the beauty that surrounds me.
Take my breath away with all of who You are–
the wonder of nature, the love of others,
and joy of family, and the taste of life.

Amen

Musical Selection

Allegro

—George Frideric Handel (1685-1759)

Chapter 16
Freedom

He is our peace. The soul is at rest. If the body follows, so be it.
This is salvation. This is freedom. This is life.

IT WAS THAT day when we went to the mall and I noticed others staring at me that it occurred to me that my life-journey had elbowed its way halfway to eternity. The fear of death and the fear of living were transformed with a bold awareness that God was my very capable Creative Director, enabling me to embrace this tragic scene in the script of my life. As long as we are afraid of death, our life will be lived in subtle bondage. Death's shadow, ominous and cold, demands respect and reverence, and apart from the resurrection of Jesus Christ, there is no hope for the great grave escape.

What is the threat of death anyway? Death threatens the loss of my physical body, true; but much more it threatens the loss of my identity. It is indeed fearsome to think that I could cease to exist or have an intellect or awareness. That thought that I might enter some eternal void where I am no longer an *ego*, a self that is uniquely me, is the most terrifying threat of death. Ironically, this very fear of death causes many to cling to life desperately, while escaping its very meaning.

Hebrews 2:14-15 reads, "Inasmuch then as the children have partaken of flesh and blood, He Himself likewise shared in the same, that through death He might destroy him who had the power of death, that is, the devil, and release those who through fear of death were all their lifetime subject to bondage." As a teenager, I would sit up on my bed and try to grasp the meaning of these verses. Someone had given me a newsletter, and these words were there in bold print. The realization that Christ's death was the transporter and transformer for the human race had never fully occurred to me before, although I had been in church for years. Christ had conquered death, and therein was the key to freedom living!

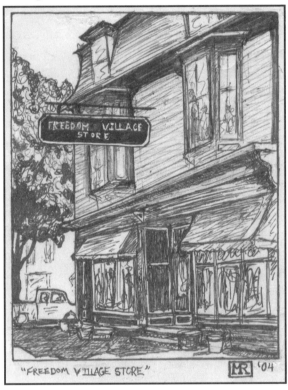

"FREEDOM VILLAGE STORE"

During much of my childhood I lived in Freedom, a tiny village in New Hampshire. Boasting a current population between 1200 and 1300, Freedom, New Hampshire, borders Maine on its east side. Freedom is named for the liberty its citizens felt after seceding from North Effingham in 1832. No one seems to know what disputes may have occurred between the folks of North Effingham and the folks of Freedom, but I've been told that the people just didn't like each other. *The Hardscrabble Chronicles*, written by Laurie Bogart Morrow, provides an intimate and alluring look at the lives of some Freedom-dwellers. I can say this: The isolation, the beauty, and the quaint country folk certainly embellish the idea of Freedom—freedom of speech or freedom from it. Some Freedom folks spoke from ignorance, others from education, and some not at all. Freedom *just to be* is what I always took it to mean.

While not in school or at 4-H meetings, most of my days in Freedom were spent hiking, sometimes barefoot, through the mountains and fields around Freedom. There was nothing that I could not and did not imagine. I was an archaeologist, digging in the woods, although the only artifacts I ever discovered were cans and bottles. I was an avid fisherman, although my catch was limited to a few minnows and bloodsuckers. I performed my operatic songs in the woods and composed tunes too dissonant to recall. I was in Freedom.

I skipped school and watched the tree-tops all day, feeling philosophical and much more intelligent for the experience. I charged honey buns at Marge's Cafe daily, since I didn't know that charge meant my parents had to pay for my taste of freedom. At recess from the two-room schoolhouse on top of the hill, I played football in fishnets because there was no choosing between the two–I was in Freedom.

Freedom in Christ is much like the village of Freedom was to me as a child. There really are no boundaries because there is total fullness in the eternal provisions of God. Freedom and fullness! God is totally satisfied with Christ's sacrifice; I have nothing valuable enough to offer that would be worthy of eternal freedom. I am free to live my life in the vastness of the liberty that Christ provided for me at a place called Calvary. Freedom from fear of death released me to fully enjoy life. God has provided freedom from self-consciousness, freedom to enjoy the divine provisions of new mercies–a return to the wonder of youthful exploration and expectation. He had provided me the freedom to rest in His peace, so that my soul is at rest. If the body follows, so be it. This is salvation. This is freedom. This is life.

Assurance that my greatest enemy–death–has been defeated is the greatest gift of all. Unwrapping this glittering box is like opening stacking boxes, except that inside each box is a new treasure, and the boxes never stop coming. I found the treasures of mercy, kindness, goodness, and faith. The treasures of peace and joy shimmer like sun-beamed raindrops. Death, the last enemy, cannot conquer our soul, for our eternal Father's open arms are filled with more treasure boxes that we can open only upon arrival at His door.

Life

Let me but live my life from year to year
With forward face and unreluctant soul,
Not hastening to, nor turning from the goal:
Not mourning for the things that disappear

In the dim past, nor holding back in fear
From what the future veils; but with a
Whole and happy heart that pays its toll
To Youth and Age, and travels on with cheer:

So let the way wind up the hill or down,
Through rough or smooth, the journey will be joy
Still seeking what I sought when but a boy
New friendship, high adventure, and a crown,
I shall grow old, but never lose life's zest.

–Henry van Dyke (1852-1933)

Today's Scripture

"Therefore, as through one man's offense judgment came to all men, resulting in condemnation, even so through one Man's righteous act the free gift came to all men, resulting in justification of life."

–Romans 5:18 (NKJV)

Quote

"I expect to pass through life but once…If therefore, there be any kindness I can show, or any good thing I can do to any fellow-being, let me do it now, and not defer or neglect it, as I shall not pass this way again."

–Stephen (Ètienne) De Grellet (1773-1855)

Prayer

Heavenly Freedom-Giver, I am ecstatic
that I have an opportunity to "pass this way."
Thank You for the freedom of living in your grace.
Amen

Musical Selection

Waltz No. 6 Db Op 64 (The Minute Waltz)
—Frederic Chopin (1810-1849)

.

Chapter 17
Freely You Have Received...
Freely Give

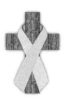

THE TIME TO do good for others is today! And you will find the blessing returned to you when you need it the most. Consider Matthew 7:12 where Jesus tells us that "...all things whatsoever ye would that men should do to you, do ye even so to them." Christianity is the only religion I know of that states this proverbial Golden Rule from the proactive perspective.

For example, Confucianism states in *Analects* 12:2, "Do not do to others what you would not like yourself. Then there will be no resentment against you, either in the family or in the state."

The *Talmud* states in *Shabbat* 3id, "What is hateful to you, do not do to your fellowman. This is the entire Law; all the rest is commentary."

Hindus are advised in *Mahabharata* 5, 1517: "This is the sum of duty; do naught unto others what you would not have them do unto you."

But Jesus is clearly telling us to move out and do something for someone! What would you want someone to do for you if you had breast cancer? Remember: The time to do for others is today. "Cast thy bread upon the waters: for thou shalt find it after many days" (Ecclesiastes 11:1).

Chapter 18
How Can I Help Thee?
Let Me Count the Ways!

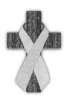

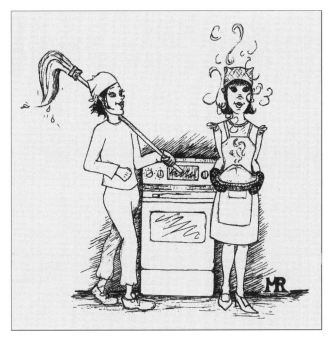

"She opens her arms to the poor and extends
her hands to the needy." (Proverbs 31:20)

IF YOU WOULD like to put the Golden Rule to work helping out your
friends or loved ones with breast cancer, here are some good ideas to get
you started.

1   Put her on your prayer list!
2   Provide a meal for the family for three days following
    chemotherapy treatments. She, the patient, probably
    doesn't even want to smell food, much less prepare it.
3   Drop off some comedy or romantic movies.

4   Pass along helpful books or periodicals about breast cancer.

5   Take the patient, your friend, out to lunch on a good day.

6   Offer to go for a walk with her; the pace may be slow–the fresh air will be great.

7   Throw a hat party–before the hair comes out.

8   Send comic strips in the mail. Dan has a sign in his office that reads, "Against the Assault of Laughter, Nothing can Stand." How true!

9   Drop by with a novel or her favorite magazines to help pass the time in waiting rooms.

10 Send a basket of lotions. Include an anti-bacterial hand cream.

11 Buy her some new make up or take her shopping; now is a great time for a new look!

12 Cozy robes and sweat suits are must-haves if the weather is cold during chemotherapy. Don't worry–she cannot have too many of either.

13 Communicate. Let her know you support her treatment decisions, even if you would have chosen something different.

14 If you happen to be a nurse or a doctor, offer to be available for weekend urgencies or concerns.

15 If you have a private vacation get-a-way spot, offer it to her and or her family. We were blessed when our friends, Harry and Kathy Hoffman, gave us their vacation home when I first heard the cancer news. We returned to the same place to celebrate two years later!

16 Buy a breast cancer awareness pin. I love mine, which my friend Kathy Hoffman gave me. I wear it proudly and often.

17 Participate in a Breast Cancer walk-a-thon on behalf of your friend.

18 Send a tempting but healthy snack basket.

19 If you work with a chemotherapy patient, help protect her from direct contact with anyone with a cold or flu.

20 Offer to clean the house. (I love this one!).

21 Send a card; it's great to receive mail when you're confined to home.

22 Send flowers; they're simply extravagant and wonderful to receive.

23 Give her a CD of soothing, relaxing music.

24 Offer to go wig shopping with her.

Chapter 19
Alternative Medicine:
Prevention & Nutrition

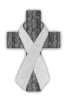

*Taking care of our bodies is a godly responsibility
and suggests that we take preventive
measures for better health.*

GENERALLY, WHEN we think of alternative medicine, we think of a treatment plan that excludes modern, conventional medical treatment. While many alternative treatments can complement the healing process, I personally did not find enough scientific confirmation to eliminate conventional treatment. I have spoken with one breast cancer survivor, however, who was revolted at the thought of chemotherapy and just couldn't bring herself to undergo the recommended treatments. Perhaps there is some truth in the idea that if you dread the treatment more than you dread the disease, then perhaps that is the wrong treatment for you.

A friend gave me a book in which a woman described her miraculous breast cancer healing. She was strongly opposed to both chemotherapy and breast cancer surgery. The author admitted that she had never had a biopsy to determine if she had breast cancer in the first place! Another man told me about a woman healed from metastasized cancer through electricity, yet further research revealed that the woman's scans had shown she never had metastasized cancer. I don't share these illustrations to dampen the enthusiasm for healing through any and all means, but I am concerned that while many fine naturopaths offer significantly helpful and beneficial healing treatments, there are perhaps a few opportunists in the mix.

On the other hand, I have uncovered a vast amount of valid information about herbs, seeds, foods, water, and air that greatly complement the healing process and can aid in the prevention of future illness. From apricot and almond seeds to wheatgrass and garlic, God has provided abundant natural resources for our health. In today's marketplace, much of what is available for the fast-food fix has preservatives, nitrates, food coloring, partially hydrogenated oils, and other DNA-damaging ingredients. Certainly a conscious effort to avoid certain known carcinogens and to eat foods known to benefit the body is a balanced and reasonable response for anyone, ill or not.

The voice of despondency and hopelessness retorts with, "I'm already ill, so what difference does it make now?" Being ill is all the more reason to focus on fortifying your natural defenses. When I became ill, I found it was the best time to make up for lost time and learn all I could about how to boost my immune system.

Taking care of our bodies is a godly responsibility and suggests that we take preventive measures for better health. My point of view is that even if I am genetically engineered not to survive beyond fifty, God may impart mercy to beat those odds, given the conscious choice of proper eating behaviors. Few people, even once they know the dangers of some foods and the healing properties of others, adhere strictly to their new way of eating. However, even small steps in the right direction may make a big difference to your future health and wellness.

Through much reading I have come to appreciate that *whole* food complements the body while chemically-altered foods tend to wreak havoc on our bodies. Since learning a bit about foods, I try to avoid chemically-altered foods, foods with antibiotics or hormones added, and foods that have been heavily treated with pesticides. As soon as I finished reading Ann Wigmore's *The Wheatgrass Book* I began taking wheatgrass each morning. During chemotherapy I had no problem with my blood counts, and I attribute that largely to the wheatgrass. I continue to take wheatgrass at least five days a week, as I believe it is one of the very best things I can do for myself. Many books have been written on the connection between nutrition and breast cancer, some of which are included in the Bibliography.

If you decide to take supportive herbs or vitamins during chemotherapy, let your doctor know what you are taking, as medicinal drugs are also derived from herbs and you will want to be sure that nothing is contraindicated. Also, I suggest making an appointment with either a naturopathic doctor or a certified herbalist to better understand what and why you are supplementing your diet. An easy mistake is to take something you don't need, or to take too much of a supplement, which could lead to adverse effects.

Another factor to consider in the healing process is the placebo effect, which means that if you truly believe that something will help you, then it probably will help you to some extent. In many cases people who were told that something would heal them were in fact healed, even though there was absolutely no scientific reason to believe that they would be. For this reason I believe that to discourage anyone from trying something they believe in would be counterproductive to that person's healing process.

My son Daniel, who is currently studying naturopathy with a concentration in Herbology at Clayton College of Natural Health, suggested the following lists of spices, herbs, plants, vegetables, fruits, protein, and carbohydrates to me. These lists are certainly not to be considered complete, as there are many other foods you can eat without guilt. What follows is a guideline to ensure that you are regularly eating at least some foods from each of these categories.

All of these are considered healing foods and can be eaten as often as you like, providing that your doctor has not advised against them. In cases where you are addressing the medical concerns of several illnesses at one time, it is always best to consult with your medical doctor first to be sure there are no contraindications. You will also find a list of rather commonly known foods to avoid, as they may be hazardous to your health!

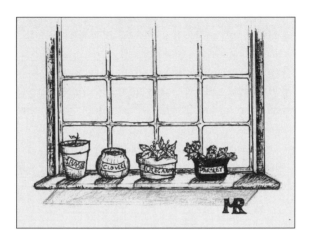

Healthy Selections

Spices, Herbs, Plants, Grasses:
Barley, barley grass, cayenne, fennel, flax meal, green tea, parsley, red clover, rosemary, sage, turmeric, wheatgrass.

Vegetables:
Apples, avocado, asparagus, beets, broccoli, brussels sprouts, cabbage, cauliflower, carrots, celery, collard greens, garlic, ginger, lima beans, onions, pea pods, peppers, pumpkin, red leaf lettuce, romaine lettuce, spinach, squash, sweet potato, tomato.

Fruits:
Apples, apricots, bananas, berries, cherries, grapes with seeds, grapefruit, grapes, lemons, melons, peaches, plums, strawberries.

Proteins:
Almonds, apricot seeds (no more than 3 at a time), black beans, chicken (organic or free-range), eggs (organic or free range), legumes, lentils, navy beans, pumpkin seeds, salmon (deep sea), sesame seeds, walnuts.

Carbohydrates:
Brown rice, corn meal, oatmeal, spinach or whole wheat pasta, whole grain cereals or breads.

Foods to Avoid

Alcohol, food coloring, luncheon meats (due to additives and nitrates), meats (beef, lamb, pork or chicken with antibiotics, hormones, or nitrates), partially hydrogenated oils, sugar.

Recipes

YOU MAY NOT feel much like cooking or eating right now, but when you do, consider a few basic recipes to get you on your way to preparing healthy foods. As a teenager, I planted a substantial vegetable garden, and with the help of friends managed to keep enough weeds away to harvest a few yummy veggies. With this garden I first discovered how delicious food is when it goes right from the ground to the mouth. Every year we experiment a little bit more with vegetables and dread when we harvest the last of the green peppers.

This year Dan and I will be trying our green thumbs at growing garlic. We are already late and will need to get it in the ground this very weekend! I am hoping to grow my own herbs indoors with the assistance of a plant light that can be purchased for a reasonable price at any hardware store.

After our growing season, we resort to the local farmers' market, a great source for fresh fruits and vegetables, many of which are not treated with pesticides. Living in Maryland, we are not far from the Pennsylvania border. So each month we take a thirty-minute drive to Shrewsbury's Amish Farmer's Market. We stock up on free-range chicken, turkey, beef, eggs, and farmer's butter. The prices are better than grocery chain prices, and the food tastes scrumptious! If you live in an area where local farmers grow their own meat organically, consider trying some. Otherwise, you can search the Internet and probably locate a source close to home.

Salad Supreme

- Broccoli
- Carrots, grated
- Cayenne pepper
- Chives
- Cucumber
- Garlic, diced
- Green pepper
- Onions
- Orange peel, organic
- Radishes
- Raw spinach leaves
- Romaine lettuce
- Shitake mushrooms
- Tomatoes

This recipe is so simple and very tasty! You can wash, chop, and mix any proportions of the above ingredients that you want. Between the cayenne (use sparingly when your stomach is sensitive), chives, and orange peel, you won't need much dressing–the flavor is already delicious. If you wish to dress it, I suggest a light vinaigrette to complement this salad that is chock-full of antioxidants and life-giving nutrients.

Sanctified Chicken Stew

- 2 gallons filtered water
- 2 pounds of boned, organic chicken thighs, chopped into 1" squares.
- ½ Head of cabbage, grated
- 5 Spring onions, chopped
- 5 Garlic cloves, chopped
- 1 Large bell pepper, chopped
- ½ Cup fresh parsley
- ¼ Cup fresh oregano
- ½ Cup barley
- 1 Tbsp. curry powder
- 2 Tsp. turmeric
- Dash of cayenne

Simply put all ingredients in a large pot and bring to a full boil. Reduce the heat to a simmer and continue cooking for about 35 minutes. Salt for more flavor, if desired.

Ham and Cabbage Soup

- 1 Hambone
- 6 Garlic cloves
- ½ Head of cabbage, grated
- 4 Stalks of celery chopped into 1" sections
- 2 Medium yellow onions, quartered
- ½ Cup of fresh oregano
- ½ Cup of fresh basil
- 1 Tbsp. fennel
- 1 Tbsp. curry
- 2 Tsp. chili powder
- 2 Tbsp. basil
- 1 Bag of frozen lima beans

Boil a hambone in 4 quarts of distilled or filtered water for 30 minutes. Remove the hambone from the water, returning the pieces of ham to the pot. Bring all of the above ingredients except the lima beans to a boil and reduce heat to a simmer. Continue to simmer for 45 minutes. Add one bag of frozen lima beans and continue to simmer for another 15 minutes. Soup may be served then, or, for enhanced flavor, refrigerate overnight and serve the follow day. Try it with cornbread.

Vegetable Medley

- 5 Turnips, cubed
- 4 Potatoes, cubed
- 8 Carrots, sliced vertically
- 5 Garlic cloves, chopped
- 3 Onions, sliced vertically
- ¼ Cup olive oil
- 3 Tbsp. fresh parsley
- 2 Tsp. cayenne
- 2 Tsp. cumin
- 2 Tsp. curry

Prepare the vegetables and put them in a baking casserole dish. In a bowl, mix the olive oil with parsley, cayenne, cumin, and curry. Drizzle this over the entire vegetable mixture and bake at 350 degrees for 45 minutes.

Spaghetti Squash Casserole

- 1 Spaghetti squash
- 3 Carrots, diced
- 4 Celery stalks, diced
- 4 Garlic cloves, minced
- 1 Large yellow onion, chopped

- 16 Oz. free range, lean ground beef
- 1 Tbsp. anise
- 1 Tbsp. nutmeg
- 2 Tsp. turmeric
- 1 Tsp. salt (optional)
- 2 Tbsp. olive oil

Boil or bake the spaghetti squash until it is cooked thoroughly and easy to remove from the skin. Mash the squash to remove any excess water; set aside. Meanwhile, sauté the carrots, celery, garlic, and onions in olive oil for 2 minutes, stirring occasionally. Add the lean ground beef and continue cooking until browned. Stir in the anise, nutmeg, turmeric, and salt (optional). Now add the spaghetti squash and stir until it is mixed in with the beef mixture. Serve with salad greens and whole wheat bread sticks, dipped in spicy olive oil.

Pernicious Penne

- 1 Tbsp. olive oil
- 3 Green peppers, cut in strips
- 5 Tomatoes, chopped into 1" chunks
- 2 Medium-sized summer squash, cut into ½" chunks

- ½ Cup of chopped walnuts3 Tbsp .flax meal
- 3 Large garlic cloves, chopped or minced
- ½ Box of whole wheat penne pasta
- Parmesan or Romano shredded cheese

Sauté the garlic and peppers in olive oil until lightly brown. Add summer squash and cook for 5 minutes, stirring occasionally. Add remaining ingredients, except the paste and cheese, and cook until tomatoes appear stewed. Meanwhile, gently boil the penne until desired texture is obtained, then strain and rinse with cool, filtered water. Serve the steaming hot vegetables over the penne and top with a generous portion of parmesan or Romano cheese. Yum!

Harvest Pasta

- 1 Tbsp. olive oil
- 3 Large garlic cloves, sliced
- 3 Green peppers, cut in strips
- 5 Tomatoes, chopped into 1" chunks
- 2 Summer squash, cut into ½" chunks
- ½ Cup chopped walnuts
- 3 Tbsp. flax meal
- 8-12 Oz. box of whole wheat penne pasta, cooked
- Parmesan cheese

Sauté garlic and peppers in olive oil until lightly brown. Add summer squash and cook for 5 minutes, stirring occasionally. Stir in remaining ingredients and cook until tomatoes appear stewed. Serve over penne pasta and top with a generous sprinkling of parmesan cheese.

Crockpot Beans and Rice

- 6 Cups of water
- ½ Pound of Northern beans
- 3 Celery stalks, chopped in 1" slices
- 5 Garlic cloves, quartered
- 1 Tbsp. turmeric
- 2 Tbsp. curry
- 2 Tbsp. Italian seasoning
- 1 Tbsp. fennel
- 1 Cup of rice

Place all the ingredients except the rice in the crockpot in the evening. In the morning, plug it in and turn it on low, stirring in the rice. When you return in the evening, you will have a delicious meal of yummy beans and rice prepared. I serve this with a Romaine lettuce salad and homemade applesauce. Oat bread will also be a nice complement to the meal for the hearty eater. I usually serve cantaloupe for dessert with this meal.

Chicken with Zucchini

- 5 Garlic cloves
- 6 Chicken thighs, skinned (organic)
- 2 Tbsp. olive oil
- 3 cups of 1" squared, chopped zucchini

Chop or press the garlic according to your preference. Skin the chicken and place along with the garlic in an electric frying pan at 350 degrees. Cover and cook for 15 minutes Turn the chicken over and add the zucchini, mixing it in with the garlic. Continue cooking for another 15 minutes for a light, delicious meal.

Steak and Peppers

- 2 Tbsp. olive oil
- 1 Red pepper, sliced vertically
- 1 Yellow pepper, sliced vertically
- 16 Oz of organic beef steak, cut into strips
- 2 Tbsp. fajita seasoning
- 1 Yellow onion, chopped
- 3 Garlic cloves, minced
- 2 Cups brown rice

Sauté peppers, onions, and garlic in the olive oil until they just begin to soften. Add the steak strips and the fajita seasoning. Continue until the meat is cooked throughout. Meanwhile, prepare enough brown rice for 4 people. Serve steak and peppers over the brown rice.

Uncle Eddie's Corn Muffins

- ½ Cup butter
- ½ Cup sugar (sugar replacement: ¼ Cup stevia or ½ Cup honey)
- 3 Eggs
- 1 Cup corn meal
- ¾ Cup white flour
- ½ Cup whole wheat flour
- ½ Tsp. baking soda
- ½ Cup soymilk
- ¾ Cup chopped dates
- ½ Cup chopped walnuts

Preheat oven to 375 degrees F. Butter and lightly flour a muffin tin. Cream together the butter and sugar. Beat the eggs separately and then stir into the creamed mixture. In a separate bowl, stir together all the dried ingredients. Then mix the flour mixture and the soymilk alternately to the creamed-egg mixture. Stir in the dates and walnuts. Bake for about 20 minutes and serve hot with butter and honey.

Yummy Yogurt Treat

- 6 Oz. vanilla yogurt (I prefer Stonyfield brand; Stonyfield guarantees the presence of multiple organisms)
- 1 Tbsp. maple syrup
- 1 Tbsp. flax meal
- 3 Tbsp. walnuts, chopped

Simply put the yogurt into the jar first, and pour on the maple syrup. Sprinkle with flax meal and walnuts and voilà! A variation of this is to blend it all together and then freeze overnight. Garnish it with crushed peppermint leaves or candy for your guests. This makes a yummy dessert

Detoxification: What, Why, & How

By Daniel R.L. Baker, B.N.H.S., N.D.

EACH DAY, whether we realize it or not, we expose ourselves to many environmental pollutants. Each person's exposure will depend on many contributing factors such as occupation, lifestyle, place of residence, and hobbies, to name a few. Environmental pollutants affect the body in many ways. Their effect can determine our bodies' oxygen assimilation levels, our ability to stay attentive, our comprehension levels, our predisposition to get cancer, and even the overall health of vital organs such as the lungs and liver.

In the lifelong process of maintaining overall good health, detoxification of the carcinogens and pollutants in the water we drink, food we eat, and air we breathe is critical in keeping all our organs capable of performing their duties at optimal levels. Detoxification is also important to keep the blood carrying as many nutrients to the cells as possible. Detoxification keeps arteries and veins all in good working order, as well as strengthening the immune system to be able to defend against invading micro-organisms and diseases. In summary, having a body in good health means having a body as free from pollutants as possible through regular detoxification.

Basic Liver Cleanse Recipe

This liver cleanse recipe is easy for anyone to follow. The doses are low to moderate and are meant to be used for adults only. Although this is a very low dose and considered safe for most adults, be sure to check for your doctor's approval before using the formula. Use only dried herbs for the following ingredients, which may be purchased at your local health food store.

- 20 Grams dandelion root
- 20 Grams echinacea
- 20 Grams reishi mushrooms
- 20 Grams yellow dock

First, dice or grind all the four herbs listed above as finely as desirable; the finer you grind them, the better the results will be. A coffee grinder works well as does a blender to obtain the desired texture. Pour the herbs into a pot and add about 1 ½ pints of cold, filtered or distilled water. Bring slowly to a boil, then decrease the heat and let the mixture simmer for 20 minutes. Allow the decoction to cool to just above room temperature, then strain the liquid using filter paper such as a coffee filter. This will provide enough for about 10 equal servings, or about 3 days' worth.

Since the dosage is about 2.4 ounces, 3 times per day, it is best to use a dropper that has ounce measurements. The quantity is so small that most people tolerate it well alone. However, if you find it bitter to the palate, you may mix it with a small amount of honey for a more appealing taste. Do not dilute it in water or juice.

Note: Dandelion root and yellow dock are "hepatic," strengthening and toning the liver. Echinacea is efficient as an immune system stimulant. Reishi mushrooms also protect the liver against damaging agents.

Radiotherapy & Breast Cancer

By Dr. Melita Braganza, M.B.B.S., D.C.H.

What Is Radiotherapy?

Radiotherapy is used to treat breast cancer, often as a back up to breast surgery. The goal of radiotherapy is to reduce the risk of cancer coming back in the healthy breast or in the lymph nodes that are treated.

Radiotherapy involves the use of radiation; it uses high energy waves to destroy the cancer cells. One may ask, "Are normal cells also affected by radiation?" Yes, they are. But they are better at repairing themselves than cancer cells.

The amount of radiotherapy prescribed depends upon the individual person's general health and the size and type of tumor. The total dose is worked out and then divided into smaller doses called 'fractions.' radiotherapy course is generally given over a number of days or weeks.

Preparing for Treatment

Before treatment is begun, radiotherapy must be planned; this means working out how much radiation the patient needs. The main objective of planning the treatment is to maximize radiation to the cancer and minimize radiation to the surrounding body tissues.

Undergoing Treatment

There are two types of radiotherapy: External Radiotherapy and Internal Radiotherapy.

External Radiotherapy is given on an outpatient basis. A machine is used to deliver the radiation, and treatment lasts for a few minutes. As treatment after breast surgery, patients typically receive radiation five times a week for at least six weeks.

Internal Radiotherapy, also called brachytherapy, is still in the experimental stage and is given on an inpatient basis. Instead of radiation from outside, radioactive substances are placed directly into the breast tissue next to the tumor. The treatment is painless and each session takes about 10 minutes.

Reactions to Radiotherapy

It is difficult to predict how a given person will react, but the following list provides some of the commonly known reactions to radioherapy.

General Reactions:

- Some people have a skin reaction, where the skin becomes red and sore like sunburn, then peels off and heals quickly. Because the skin may become more sensitive, loose-fitting clothes and a high factor sun screen are often advised.

- Treatment can make a person feel sick and cause some weight loss due to loss of appetite. An anti-nausea medication is generally prescribed, which is taken prior to the treatment.

- Some people may develop a cough or shortness of breath that generally lasts a few days.

- Fatigue can also be a side-effect.

- Radiation may also cause a reduction in white blood cells.

Long-term Side-Effects:

- Skin may look darker and feel different to the touch.

- Red spidery marks may appear from small broken blood vessels.

- Healthy tissues can become less stretchy–the breast may feel different.

- Drainage channels to the arms may become blocked causing swelling of the upper limbs.

Why Is Radiotherapy Used?

Radiotherapy may be used as any of these types of treatment:

- *Curative treatment*–to destroy the tumor and cure cancer.
- *Palliative treatment*–to relieve symptoms and reduce pain
- *Neo adjuvant treatment*–to shrink the tumor and reduce the risk of spreading during surgery.
- *Adjuvant treatment*–to kill any cancer cells that have been left after surgery.

Dr. Melita Braganza has been a primary care pediatrician in India for several years. She has also lived in Auckland, New Zealand for five years where she continued working as a physician. She currently lives in Baltimore with her husband. She is working in medical research and coordinates clinical trials at both the Vascular Surgery division of the University of Maryland Hospital and the VA Medical Center. She has a passion for research and finds working with the veterans most rewarding. Her family includes three children and five grandchildren.

Chemotherapy

By Dr. N. Joseph Haroun, M.D.

Chemotherapy is a term that refers to the treatment of cancer with drugs that can destroy cancer cells. There are a variety of ways that these anti-cancer drugs can be given, which include intravenously by injection, intravenously by pump or in pill form, taken by mouth.

How Does Chemotherapy Work?

The normal cells in our bodies are programmed to grow and die in a controlled way. However, when abnormal cells divide and form new cells without control, the result is cancer. The anti-cancer drugs prevent cancer cells from growing or multiplying. Each drug works against a specific cancer and there are specific doses and schedules for taking each one. Some drugs work more effectively when used together than they do when used alone. Thus, "combination therapy" is used, which means two or more drugs are given at the same time.

Other types of drugs can be used to treat your cancer. For instance, some drugs can block the effects of your body's hormones. Then there is biological therapy, which is a treatment with substances to boost the body's immune system against the cancer.

What Are the Goals of Chemotherapy?

Chemotherapy is used to reach different goals, depending on the type of cancer and how advanced it is. The first goal would be to cure the cancer and is evidenced when the patient remains free of cancer cells. Secondly, chemotherapy can control cancer by keeping it from spreading and by slowing its growth. It also kills cancer cells that may have spread to other parts of the body from the cancer's place of origin. Another goal would be to alleviate symptoms caused by cancer and bring comfort to the patient.

What Are the Side-Effects of Chemotherapy?

Unfortunately, healthy cells can be harmed by chemotherapy, especially those that divide quickly. Some examples are the membranes that line the mouth, the lining of the gastrointestinal tract, the hair follicles, and the bone marrow. Side-effects occur because of the damage to these healthy cells. Side-effects of chemotherapy may include:

- Nausea and vomiting
- Loss of appetite
- Hair loss
- Mouth sores
- Diarrhea
- Rash on hands and feet
- Increased risk of infection
- Bleeding and bruising easily from minor injuries
- Fatigue related to anemia

When chemotherapy is stopped, the sideeffects will go away, though it may take some time. The patient should always communicate any side-effects to the treating physician, as these effects can be alleviated or prevented with medications or a change in diet.

Dr. Naji Haroun graduated from the American University of Medical School in Beirut. He received his training in internal medicine at Rutgers University Medical School in New Jersey. Dr. Haroun received his post doctoral fellowship training in endocrinology at Johns Hopkins in Baltimore, Maryland. Since that time he has been in private practice in Baltimore, Maryland.

Tamoxifen the "Wonder Drug"

By Dr. Chris Wright, Ph.D.

What Are Oestrogens?

Oestogens (estrogens) are potent steroidal hormones made naturally in the body by the ovaries in pre-menopausal, non-pregnant women. Their chemical structure is similar to all steroid hormones, biologically derived from cholesterol. Production of steroids in the female occurs principally in the adrenal cortex and ovaries. Only three oestrogens are found in significant quantities in the female: oestrdiol, oestrone, and oestriol. B-oestradiol, the principal oestrogen secreted by the ovaries, is considered to be the major oestrogen.

What Do Oestrogens Do?

The principal function of the oestrogens is to cause cellular proliferation and growth of the tissues of the sexual organs and of other tissues related to reproduction, including mammary glands and the uterus. The proliferation and growth of tissue becomes a concern when cancer is present.

How Do Oestrogens Work?

As previously mentioned, oestrogens are steroidal compounds, like the fat soluble vitamin D. This chemical property of the molecule allows them to enter cells with ease since they can pass through the cell membrane and gain access to the nucleus of the cell. Oestrogen works, like other hormones, by switching on genes in their target cell. Genes are short sequences of DNA, the cell's code and instructions for making new products. Once inside a cell, oestrogen binds with a specific receptor, triggering a gene into action. The final result of this is cell division.

The History of Anti-Oestrogens

Early synthetic anti-oestrogens were known to have oestrogenic as well as anti-oestrogenic properties, and this prompted the search for developing more anti-oestrogen compounds. Tamoxifen soon became a front runner, first known as "Nolvadex." Its effective dose of 10-20 mg reported clearly low toxicity. Like many biological systems that God created, the tamoxifen story is incredibly complex. Initially, the pharmacological effects of tamoxifen were confusing: laboratory tests showed it to behave as a pure oestrogen, partial oestrogen, or as an anti-oestrogen, depending on the tissue and the species studied. These various tissues include breast tissue, the endometrium, and bone tissue.

Breast Cancer Treatment Options

Links between exposure to oestrogens and cancer, endogenous (natural, within the body), or exogenous (the contraceptive pill, for example) have caused controversial debate for many years. Thus, some form of endocrine therapy seemed an obvious option for treatment. This therapy has mainly been achieved by:

a) Indirectly reducing the supply of oestrogens to the cells.

b) Direct interaction with the oestrogen receptor.

The option selected depends on menopausal status. For premenopausal women, a reduction in the circulating levels of oestrogens may be achieved surgically by oophorectomy (removal of the ovaries), first recognized as early as 1889 as a treatment for breast cancer. Alternatively, irradiation of the ovaries has been used to artificially induce menopause. However, some endogenous oestrogens still exist due to what is called "peripheral aromatization" of androstenedione. This occurs naturally in post-menopausal women when the body's fatty tissues convert the hormone androstenedione, (a hormone derived from cholesterol, similar to the male sex hormone testosterone,) to oestrone. Oestrone may then be converted to the active oestrogen oestradiol which binds with the oestrogen receptor. Approximately 70% of the androstenedione is produced by the adrenal glands. Thus, previous methods of treatment have been aimed at reducing or inhibiting the aromatase enzymes (chemical catalysts within cells) which are responsible for making the peripheral oestrogens. While surgical removal of the adrenal glands was added to the drastic measures taken by early attempts to treat breast cancer, treatment with drugs designed to inhibit the aromatase enzymes proved to be a logical approach with some success.

One of the main glands in the body which orchestrates many hormonal responses is the pituitary gland, situated in the brain. The pituitary gland controls levels of Follicle Stimulation Hormone and Luteinising Hormone which, in turn, control oestrogen levels in pre-menopausal women. Past treatments investigated have included surgical removal of the pituitary gland and drugs to block release of the chemical messengers from the pituitary gland, which stimulate oestrogen production. Believe it or not, large doses of oestrogen have been used to treat breast cancer! Prior to the introduction of tamoxifen, diethystiboestrol, a synthetic oestrogen, was widely used as first-line endocrine therapy in postmenopausal women with advanced breast cancer. Many of the treatments outlined above have unwanted side-effects: surgical removal of glands depletes the body of other natural secretions, while drugs can have numerous side-effects.

How Does Tamoxifen Work?

Tamoxifen is described as a non-steroidal, synthetic anti-oestrogen, similar in structure to B-oestradiol, the major oestrogen. Tamoxifen is made in the laboratory by pharmaceutical companies. Because its molecular structure is so similar to that of B-oestradiol, it binds with the oestrogen receptor in cells. A simple analogy for this reaction between a molecule and a receptor is a "lock and key." The receptor behaves as a lock, and the molecule behaves as the key. Keys are very specific for their locks, and lock will only turn if the right key is inserted. If a similar key is inserted in the lock, it will block the hole for the "correct" key, but will not turn the lock to open the door or fixture. In the same manner, tamoxifen binds with oestrogen receptors, due to its similarity in structure to B-oestradiol, and blocks naturally produced oestrogens from binding.

Tamoxifen–The New Wonder Drug!

Research and trial and error with various treatments heralded tamoxifen as the new wonder drug to treat breast cancer. Prompted by the discovery of anti-oestrogenic actions of tamoxifen in rats in 1967, researchers conducted a clinical trial in 1971 indicating that about one-fifth of patients showed a good response. The effectiveness of tamoxifen was subsequently analyzed in a number of clinical trials throughout the 1980s. Based on results involving 75,000 women–30,000 treated with tamoxifen and 26,000 with chemotherapy only–highly significant and similar reductions in annual rates of recurrence and death were found.

Side-Effects of Tamoxifen

The most frequent adverse effects are related to the drug's anti-oestrogenic activity and include hot flashes, nausea and/or vomiting, vaginal bleeding, or discharge, and menstrual disturbances. One of the main concerns is the uncertainty over the effect of tamoxifen on the endometrium (uterus) and the liver. A number of studies suggest that tamoxifen does exert an oestrogen effect on the endometrium and may increase the risk of endometrial cancer.

Note: Raloxifene, a more recently developed anti-oestrogen, related to tamoxifen, is currently undergoing trials (U.S. National Cancer Institute STAR trial) and is being compared to tamoxifen. It is thought that raloxifene may not have an oestrogenic effect on the endometrium.

Effects of Oestrogen and Tamoxifen on Bone

There was initially a concern that long-term tamoxifen therapy might increase bone loss at times in pre-menopausal women, thus increasing the risk and incidence of fractures. Bone is a living tissue and changes throughout one's life. After the age of 30, there is a natural age-related decrease in bone mass. There is a clear link between oestrogen status and maintenance of bone mass in women. When oestrogen levels naturally fall after menopause, extensive studies have shown that there is an increase in the rate of bone loss resulting in reduced bone mass.

As you are probably aware, if you break a bone, it mends; a new piece of bone grows between two fractured ends and knits it together. Once bone has been made it is constantly remodeled in order to maintain strength. This is achieved by a simple cycle involving bone cells called osteoclasts and osteoblasts. The osteoclasts literally erode away the old bone, whilst the osteoblasts make new bone tissue that is hardened with calcium. The extent to which the osteoclasts erode old bone is thought to be under the control of oestrogen. In the absence of oestrogen, more erosion takes place–hence, the initial concern about tamoxifen therapy increasing bone loss in pre-menopausal women.

Well, rest assured. One of the first clinical trials of its type in the world conducted at Cambridge University, UK, investigated the effect of long-term tamoxifen therapy on bone remodeling and structure in women with breast cancer. This work formed the basis for my Ph.D. thesis and was published in the *British Medical Journal* in 1993. It concluded that tamoxifen does not have an adverse effect and, if anything, has a slight positive effect on bone! So the wonder drug not only protects against breast cancer, but may even be good for your skeleton, too!

After studying for a MS in Toxicology at Surrey University, Dr. Chris Wright gained his Ph.D. from Cambridge University, England, while working at Addenbrookes Hospital as a research scientist. His research was sponsored by the Cancer Research Campaign (UK) and supervised by Dr. Juliet Compston, a high respected and well-published authority on osteoporosis and metabolic bone dis-

ease at Cambridge University. Together, Dr. Wright and Dr. Compston carried out the first unique in vivo study of the effect of long term tamoxifen therapy on postmenopausal women with breast cancer. The results of their comprehensive investigation were published in the British Medical Journal in 1993. Chris is currently Head of Biology at Archbishop Tenison's Church of England Secondary School in London. Chris is a Christian, a keen outdoor enthusiast and married with two children. He hopes that this book will bring comfort and relief to breast cancer sufferers worldwide and he thanks God that he had the opportunity to carry out the invaluable research on tamoxifen.

References & Reading

Sources

Beyond the Shock: A Step by Step Guide to the Diagnosis of Breast Cancer. Interactive CD for patients written by doctors. (MedEd Distribution.) Proceeds of these sales go directly to provide mammograms to women unable to afford this important screening procedure and to further breast cancer education.

National Breast Cancer Organization. www.nationalbreastcancer.org/signs_and_symptoms/index.html

A Breast Cancer Journey: Your Personal Guidebook (2nd Edition). American Cancer Society, 2004.

Suggested Reading

Bacon, Richard M. *The Forgotten Art of Growing, Gardening, and Cooking with Herbs.* (Dublin, NH: Yankee, Inc., 1972.)

Benjamin, Harold H. *The Wellness Community Guide to Fighting for Recovery from Cancer.* (New York: Penguin Putnam Inc., 1995.)

Egoscue, Pete. *Pain Free: A Revolutionary Method for Stopping Chronic Pain.* (New York: Bantam, 1998.)

Jensen, Bernard. *Dr. Jensen's Guide to Better Bowel Care.* (New York: Avery, 1999.)

Morrow, Laurie Bogart. *The Hardscrabble Chronicles.* (New York: Berkley Books, 2002.)

Nash, Jennie. *The Victoria's Secret Catalogue Never Stops Coming.* (New York: Simon and Schuster, 2001.)

Slaga, Thomas. *The Detox Revolution.* (New York: McGraw-Hill, 2003.)

Seibold, Ronald L. *Cereal Grass: What's in it For You.* (Lawrence, Kansas. Wilderness Community Education Foundation, Inc., 1990.)

Weil, Andrew, and Daley, Rosie. *The Healthy Kitchen*. (New York: Random House, 2002.)

Bibliography

Arnot, Robert. *The Breast Cancer Prevention Diet*. (Boston, NY, London: Little, Brown and Company, 1998.)

Bruss, Katherine and Sproull, Amy. *A Breast Cancer Journey*. (Atlanta, GA: American Cancer Society, 2001.)

Colbert, Don. *The Bible Cure for Cancer*. (Florida: Siloam Press, 1999.)

Dubin, Reese. *Miracle Food Cures from the Bible*. (New Jersey: Prentice Hall Press, 1999.)

Felleman, Hazel. *The Best Loved Poems of the American People*. (New York: Double Day, 1936).

Hatherill, Robert. *Eat to Beat Cancer*. (Los Angeles, CA: Renaissance Books, 1998.)

Hay, Louise. *You Can Heal Your Life*. (Carlsbad, CA: Hay House, Inc., 1987.)

Knight, Walter. *Master Book of New Illustrations*. (Wm. B. Eerdmans Publishing Co., 1994.)

Morgan, Robert J. *Nelson's Complete Book of Stories, Illustrations, and Quotes: The Ultimate Contemporary Resource for Speakers*. (Nashville, Tennessee. Thomas Nelson, Inc., 2000.)

Siegel, Bernie. *Peace, Love, and Healing*. (New York: Harper and Row Publishers, Inc., 1998.)

The Harvard Classics, English Poetry in Three Volumes. Volume III. (New York: P.F. Collier and Son Corporation, 1938.)

Weil, Andrew. *Natural Health, Natural Medicine*. (New York: Houghton Mifflin Company, 1998.)

Wigmore, Anne. *The Wheatgrass Book*. (New Jersey: Avery Publishing Group, Inc., 1985.)

Cancer Resources

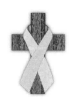

American Cancer Society
800-ACS-2345
www.cancer.org

AMC Harford County
P.O. Box 933
Bel Air, MD 21014
www.amc.org

American Institute for Cancer Research
202-328-7744
www.aicr.org

Cancer Survivors Network
877-333-4673 (HOPE)
www.cancer.org

Cancer Information Counseling Line (CICL)
800-525-3777
www.amc.org

Corporate Angel Network
914-328-1313
www.corpangelnetwork.org

Hospice Cares
www.hospice-cares.com

National Alliance of Breast Cancer Organizations
212-719-4154
www.charitynavigator.org

National Cancer Institute
800-4-CANCER
www.nci.nih.gov

National Cancer Survivors Day Foundation (NSCD)
615-791-4719
www.ncsdf.org

Susan B. Komen Breast Cancer Foundation
800-462-9273
www.komen.org

The Breast Cancer Site
www.thebreastcancersite.com

The Wellness Community
310-314-2555
www.thewellnesscommunity.org

Womens's Information Network Against Breast Cancer
866-294-6222
www.winabc.org

Y-ME National Breast Cancer Organization
800-221-2141
www.y-me.org

About the Author

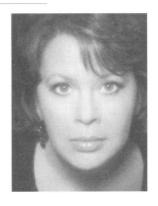

SYLVIA MORGAN BAKER has, for the past eleven years, co-labored with her husband Dan L. Baker at a diversely populated private school in Baltimore, Maryland, where she serves as the elementary principal and dean of curriculum development.

When she was diagnosed with breast cancer, Sylvia began to look in earnest for God's promises and provisions so that she would not be robbed of her usual joyful and optimistic outlook on life. Two years later, she is writing about the experience and the many facets of beauty and grace that she discovered in unexpected trials.

Sylvia has a Master's degree in Education Administration and has been honored by the Congressional Youth Leadership Council for her guidance and leadership among today's youth. She also holds a lifetime Professional Elementary Principal Certification from the Association of the Christian Schools International. She now hopes to bring spiritual guidance, comfort, and joy to women everywhere who have breast cancer, or may have to face its challenges in the future. Recently her elementary teachers gave her a card that depicts her firecely determined spirit with the inscription: "We will either find a way or make one."

Sylvia has been a featured speaker at the Indianapolis Women's Conference and the Greater Grace International Women's Convention. She has written and taught a course for high school seniors entitled Christian Ethics and Apologetics. Sylvia speaks frequently to high school students about issues relevant to spiritual growth and how establishing the mind in God's thoughts leads to positive emotions. Since recovering from breast cancer, she supports women who are fighting the good fight against this dreaded disease in any way that she can, including American Cancer Society fund-raising projects, Reach to Recover, and Tell A Friend programs.